THE ETHICS OF SUFFERING

The Ethics of Suffering presents an accessible introduction to philosophical and ethical issues raised by the legal regulation of medical practice. Examining case studies in medical law and medical ethics in both the English and North American contexts, this book explores the suffering involved in controversial legal cases such as euthanasia, withdrawal of life-support from comatose patients, treating elderly patients without consent, and sterilisation of incompetent patients.

Focusing on the concept of suffering in medicine and law, this book engages the law with the central philosophical notions of Lévinas to explore the interiority and suffering that structures the doctor-patient relationship. The book, further, highlights the negative consequences of law's reluctance to pose questions related to the subjective and often irrational responses to human suffering.

Diamantides offers a powerful critique of the legal concepts of patients' rights and interests, and suggests a radical rewriting of the theory of justice as it applies to medical law. Presenting an original and accessible study in an area of expanding importance and interest for lawyers, philosophers and place makers, this book crosses a number of conventional boundaries between disciplines and professions, and will be of wide interest to students, researchers and professionals alike.

ASHGATE STUDIES IN APPLIED ETHICS

Scandals in medical research and practice; physicians unsure how to manage new powers to postpone death and reshape life; business people operating in a world with few borders; unprofessional conduct in scientific research; damage to the environment; concern regarding the welfare of animals - all have prompted an international demand for ethical standards which go beyond matters of personal taste and opinion.

The *Ashgate Studies in Applied Ethics* series presents leading international research on the most topical areas of applied and professional ethics, recognizing that the revival of interest in applied ethics is a return to an important role for philosophers: a concern with justice and good conduct in all spheres of life. Focusing particularly on professional, business, environmental, medical and bio-ethics, the series draws from many diverse interdisciplinary perspectives including: philosophical, historical, legal, medical, environmental and sociological. Exploring the intersection of theory and practice, books in this series will prove of particular value to researchers, students, and practitioners worldwide.

Series Editors:

Ruth Chadwick, Head of Centre for Professional Ethics & Professor of Moral
Philosophy, University of Central Lancashire, UK
David Lamb, Honorary Reader in Bioethics, University of Birmingham, UK
Michael Davis, Center for the Study of Ethics in the Professions,
Illinois Institute of Technology, USA

The Ethics of Suffering
Modern law, philosophy and medicine

MARINOS DIAMANTIDES

Ashgate

Aldershot • Burlington USA • Singapore • Sydney

Published by
Ashgate Publishing Ltd
Gower House
Croft Road
Aldershot
Hants GU11 3HR
England

Ashgate Publishing Company
131 Main Street
Burlington, VT 05401-5600 USA

Ashgate website: http://www.ashgate.com

British Library Cataloguing in Publication Data
Diamantides, Marinos
    The ethics of suffering : modern law, philosophy and
    medicine. - (Ashgate studies in applied ethics)
    1. Suffering - Moral and ethical aspects
    I. Title
    179.7

Library of Congress Control Number: 00-133528

ISBN 0 7546 1326 7

Printed and bound by Athenaeum Press, Ltd.,
Gateshead, Tyne & Wear.

THANK GOODNESS

Contents

We think that beyond the apparent negativity of the idea of the Infinite, one can and must find the forgotten horizons of its abstract signification; one must bring the reversal of teleology of the act of consciousness in disinterested thought back to the non-fortuitous conditions and circumstances of its signifying in humankind, whose humanity is, perhaps, the putting back into question of the good conscience of being that perseveres in being; and it is advisable to reconstitute the indispensable scenery of the 'staging' of this reversal.

Emmanuel Lévinas

Time and the Other transl. Richard A. Cohen
Duquesne University Press Pittsburgh Pennsylvania 1987: 135

Preface

Philosophically, this book aims to express a simple, if forgotten, truth which is expressed in the philosophical work of Emmanuel Lévinas: justice (be it state justice or informal one) is not possible without the one that renders it finding himself caught in proximity. However, 'proximity' in its ethical sense is not to be confused with the enjoyment of inter-subjective contiguity, co-presence or convergence and, hence, is not absent in situations of formal abstraction. Instead, 'affective proximity' emerges in response to separation, loss and witnessing of absurd suffering in others.

The main epistemological premise is that the source of meaningful society is not intentionality and utility but 'unintentional affectivity' of one being for another. From such purely emotional rapports, which control even relationships that are seemingly based only on knowledge or kinship, stem the anarchic vocations of solidarity and compassion which seek to respond to the absurdity of human suffering as witnessed in the face of the other being. The meaningfulness of our collective social organization must be sought in relation to our lived feelings of responsibility for one another, even though affectivity comes unintentionally (i.e. before the ego emerges) and anarchically (that is not due to law but for the sake of justice). Nevertheless, such individuated responsibility is experienced as an obsession and exercised as a vocation. The modern subject of law finds itself in a dilemma: either to be seen as acting 'irresponsibly' or to obscure its individuated responsibility by means of falsely 'objective' truths and justifications.

In this light the book examines various situations arising in the context of medical law and medical ethics in both the English and North American contexts. Looking closely at the suffering involved in controversial legal cases of euthanasia, withdrawal of life-support from comatose patients, treating elderly patients without consent and sterilisation of incompetent patients, the book engages the law with some of Emmanuel Lévinas's key notions. These include 'affectivity', 'proximity' and the 'vocation of compassion' that is activated as humans witness the 'absurdity' of suffering. Along the way the book asserts that the moral difficulty with many contemporary medico-legal issues is not due to the specificity of the facts nor the impropriety of the normative framework. The problem, rather, lies with the irresponsibility of the relevant decision-makers for the 'affectivity' and 'ethical violence' of their decisions. In law, particularly, this irresponsibility often mars judicial decisions with false justifications causing them to act later as bad precedents. The language in which modern legal judgments are justified is so structured that the sense of affective proximity with the patient is lost and affectivity is perversely connected with irresponsibility. This renders human rights claims by lawyers and judges unintelligible in an ethical context since human rights are not understood as a form of compassion as they ought to be. In ethical terms justice to the sufferer requires an emotional rapport and an overwhelming sense of responsibility which acts as a background in front of which alone can the absurdity and incommensurability of human suffering be acknowledged. Without an emotional rapport with the patient it is impossible to 'stage' suffering and responsibility in their entirety, and doctors and judges are resigned to representing them elliptically and selectively. This gives rise to a comprehensive critique of such pivotal elements of medico-legal doctrine as 'informed consent', 'percentage of risk', 'best interests test', 'test of competency', 'double effect doctrine', the perceived moral difference between active and passive euthanasia, the distinction between 'ordinary and extraordinary treatment' etc.

Moreover the book attempts to explain the general aspects of judicial policy in relation to patients and doctors. Why are judges reluctant to criminalise medical therapeutic interventions without the patient's informed consent? Why are the standards for successful medical suits constantly maximised directly or indirectly? Why, overall, do judges send the message that informal dispute resolution is preferable for doctor-patient disputes? The novelty of the book is that in relation to these matters it does not take a black-letter legal approach whereby the problems are strictly to do with misapplication of doctrine. Nor is the book's main intention to seek through these examples to show the regulatory symbiosis between post-sovereignty law and modern medicine in circumstances of bio-politics. The purpose, rather, is to show that the inappropriate use of legal doctrine and the political instrumentalisation of medicine can only occur effectively in conditions in which both the legal and medical practices are ethically disorientated. In law the disorientation occurs due to the legal doctrine's aversion to engage with natural 'suffering'. Thus, the problematic policies mentioned above are explained in relation to the inability of judges to account for their affectivity in relation to the human rights of suffering patients. Under modern auspices, the medico-legal judgment must focus exclusively on man-caused 'harm' and has little to say for 'naturally' inflicted suffering. And yet, it is here argued, it is in relation to responsibility for 'suffering that no-one has caused' that all notions of responsibility emerge philosophically.

In more theoretical terms, the book aims to become a first step towards an innovative and accessible 'jurisprudence of suffering' which would offer an alternative starting point to the student or researcher of medico-legal ethics and which would necessarily contrast with the vast majority of the existing literature.

On the one hand, medical law textbooks concentrate on the piecemeal judicial attempts to cover doctor-patient disputes by expanding traditional criminal and tort law doctrines which are built around the notions of assault and harm. My book, by contrast, takes as its starting point the notion of ethical responsibility for natural suffering and depicts the degree to which the doctrinal approach needs to be re-evaluated. In this respect, the book systematically develops a proper 'jurisprudence of suffering' which gives central place to the individual vocations of gratuitous affectivity and compassion for 'absurd' suffering. On the other hand, there is a large literature in medical sociology of the Foucaultian legacy which concentrates on modern governance and the state's interest in regulating life increasingly through the medium of medicine and, decreasingly, through legal norms. In response to this the book shows the jurisprudence of suffering simultaneously to complement Foucault's approach and to stand independently of it. For in the ethics promoted here the centrality given to the individual's capacity to be affected by 'absurd' suffering goes hand in hand with a capacity to remain 'disinterested' in those 'facts' of individual life which constitute the pivotal element of a bio-politics. In this connection the book argues, additionally, that the modern state's interest in individual lives has also necessitated the legal institutionalisation of ethical indifference towards incurable suffering most notably by means of representing certain situations as 'marginal', 'extraordinary', 'excessive', 'exceptional' and so on. This is shown not only in the resistance of common law to the civil 'duty to provide assistance' but, also, in all the key-notions of English and American medico-legal doctrine examined in the book. Finally, a synthetic argument emerges regarding the moral consequences for the individual in the Western juridico-political order from the legal suppression of the ethics of suffering and the institution of self-care and moral indifference.

Introduction

The human *esse* is not *conatus* but disinterestedness and *a-dieu* (MT: 25).[1]

If ethical terms arise in our discourse before the terms 'freedom' and 'non-freedom', it is because before the bipolarity of good and evil is presented to choice, the subject finds himself committed to the Good in the passive [role] of the *supporter* of the entire universe. To support the universe is a crushing charge but also a divine discomfort (OB: 122).

Justice consists in making possible expression [in circumstances of] ... non-reciprocity [whereby] ... the person presents himself as unique. Justice is a right to speak (TaI: 298).

Even ... in [a] climate of uniformity, it is possible to express the exceptional ethical significance of a particular Saying producing itself as *me* and capable of repetition, that is of re-producing itself as me time after time, again and again. In the dimension of the Said the meaning of such a situation becomes universal, while its unsayable Saying precedes the Said and lies in the ipseity of the subject in the Saying. Faced with the Saying and the Said, we should not make the mistake of looking for too rigid a hierarchical relation between the two orders. In fact their interdependency and the fluctuation between them open an endless field of ambiguity with reference to subjectivity. In *Otherwise than Being* Lévinas deliberately courts this ambiguity in order to preserve the particularity of the subject alongside its universal ethical significance. The ambiguity allows Lévinas to speak and to write of both of these possibilities in the dislocation of a diachronic thought. He thinks 'a thought that is one but not thought at the same time' [*pensée une, mais non pensée en même temps*] (F. Ciaramelli in Bernasconi and Critchley, eds. 1991: 93).

I
The premises: ethics, proximity, law

ETHICS Let me say a few things about the title of this thesis, beginning with what I mean by 'ethical'. Today 'ethics' may mean little to those who find that, in post-

---

[1] All titles of books by Emmanuel Lévinas are cited in an abbreviated form: see the Bibliography for key to these abbreviations.

modernity, we have finally entered the 'post-duty, post-deontic epoch, where our conduct has been freed from the last vestiges of oppressive "infinite duties", "commandments" and "absolute obligations"'.[2] For others, however, the above views are only partly true. On the one hand, it is true that we are today experiencing the demise of modern ethical thought. Modern ethical thought had attempted - but failed - to devise a 'cohesive code of moral rules which people could be taught and forced to obey - in "co-operation with legislative practice"' (Zygmunt Bauman 1993: 6). On the other hand, Bauman also observes, it is *not* true that this demise is the symptom, as is often believed, of an era in which, supposedly,

> people grew individually minded, self-concerned and egotistic, as with the advent of modernity they became godless and lost their faith in 'religious dogmas' (Bauman 1993: 5).

Rather, the cause of the failure is to be found within the attempt to 'codify/rationalise ethics' (Bauman 1993: 6). This occurred in the aftermath of the advent of secularism and was the result of the predominant philosophy of the Enlightenment. First:

> modern legislators and modern thinkers alike felt that morality, rather than being a 'natural trait' of human life, is something that needs to be designed and injected into human conduct ... They earnestly believed that ... *reason* can do what *belief* [in God] was doing no more; that with their eyes open and passions put to rest, men can regulate their mutual relationships no less, and perhaps more and better (in a more 'civilised', peaceful, rational manner) than at a time when they were blinded by faith and when their untamed and undomesticated feelings ran wild (ibid. 6-7).

Moreover, second:

> [W]hen viewed 'from the top' by those responsible for the 'running of society' ... [The individual's] untoward, potentially heinous impulses needed to be held in check - either from inside or from the outside: either by the actors themselves, through the exercise of their 'better judgement' suppressing their instincts with the help of their rational faculties - or through exposing the actors to rationally designed external pressures which would assure that 'doing wrong does not pay' and so most individuals most of the time are discouraged from doing it (ibid.).

Indeed, in the west we passed from the Christian preconception of the human being as 'fallen angel' to the modern one in which the human was thought to be 'naturally' immoral, and now, to one which effectively accuses the individual once again of godlessness - although this time in a tragically ironic sense, with the

---

[2]From Gilles Lipovetsky, *Le Crépuscule du devoir*, as cited in Bauman 1993: 6.

cynicism of the one who remarks that 'even if there is no God we have to invent one'. For Bauman, however, if modern ethical thought 'failed' in the end to conjure and enforce a 'universal' and 'codified' substantive morality - as promised - this 'failure' must be seen as 'inherent' in modernity's project. This, I submit, takes the form of a principle of procrastination, of deferral of the accomplishment of all that the project of humanism intended. In Bauman's words again:

> the persevering and unyielding search for rules that 'will stick' and foundations that 'won't shake' drew its animus from the faith in the feasibility and ultimate triumph of the humanist project. A society free from irrevocable contradictions, a society pointing the way, as logic does, to correct solutions only, can be built eventually, given enough time and good will ... In other words, the moral thought and practice of modernity was animated by a belief in the possibility of a non-ambivalent, non-aporetic code. Perhaps such a code has not been found yet. But it surely waits round the corner. Or the corner after next ... (ibid. 9).

Bauman, moreover, succinctly states how those same forces which sought to 'inject' the individual with morality - not least by controlling the relationship of the individual to him or herself through teaching and instruction as to how to suppress one's moral impulses - also unleashed the potential for the downfall of the modern aspiration to create, and enforce, moral rationalism and uniformity. As he observes (making implicit reference to Michel Foucault's hermeneutics of the subject):

> Developing individual powers of judgement (training individuals to see what is in their interest and to follow their interest once they saw it) and managing the stakes in such a fashion that pursuit of individual interest would prompt them to obey the order the legislators wished to install, had to be seen as conditioning and complementing each other; they made sense only together. On the other hand, however, they were potentially at cross-purposes. 'From the top' the individual judgement could never look completely reliable and this simply for the fact of being individual and thus rooted in an authority *other than* that of the guardians and spokesmen of order...Autonomy of rational individuals and heteronomy of rational management were likely to resent and resist interference (ibid. 7; my emphasis).

More generally, in presenting modernity's moral programmatic failure not as a 'failure', but as consequence of modernity's disdain of 'individual judgement...rooted in an authority other than one found in the order itself, Bauman shows the skill of a post-modern ethicist that I wish to emulate in this thesis. Bauman's words below express to a degree my own approach to ethics:

> the novelty of the post-modern approach to ethics consists first and foremost *not* in the abandoning of characteristically modern moral concerns, but in the rejection of the typically modern ways of going about its moral problems (that is, responding to

moral challenges with coercive normative regulation in political practice, and the philosophical search for absolutes, universals and foundations in theory). The great issues of ethics - like human rights, social justice, balance between peaceful co-operation and personal self-assertion, synchronisation of individual conduct and collective welfare - have lost nothing of their topicality. They only need to be seen and dealt with in a novel way (ibid. 4).

Although I wish to emulate Bauman's style - the style of an ethicist who celebrates the lack of feasibility of a comprehensive 'moral code' which would be universally meaningful - I will, however, promptly take leave of Bauman's overall rejection of the search for 'universals'. The ethical philosophy of Emmanuel Lévinas which inspires this thesis equips me to take just such an approach, which I explain below under 'proximity'. Let me, however, conclude this section on ethics in post-modern times with a summary of Bauman's 'seven marks of moral condition' as they appear once contemplated from a post-modern perspective (which I will promptly qualify) (Bauman 1993: 10-15). These are (one) that humans 'are morally ambivalent' and (two) rationality cannot 'override moral impulse', and (three) that all subsequent 'social arrangements, the power-assisted institutions as well as the rationally articulated and pondered rules and duties, deploy that ambivalence as their building material while doing their best to cleanse it from its original sin of being an ambivalence'. Bauman's fourth point generalises that moral phenomena are 'inherently non-rational', and that morality is 'incurably aporetic' and 'not universalizable'. Given the ambiguous impacts of the societal efforts at ethical legislation one must assume that (five) 'moral responsibility, being *for* the other before one can be *with* the other, is the first reality of the self, a starting point rather than a product of society'. And (six) morality 'has no excuse', because it precedes the emergence of the 'socially administered context inside which the terms in which justifications and excuses ... make sense. That question demands that morality show the certificate of its origin - *yet* there is no self before the moral self ...'.[3]

---

[3] In these circumstances, Bauman adds as his seventh point: 'the post-modern perspective on moral phenomena does not reveal the relativism of morality. Neither must it call for ... disarmament in the face of an apparently irreducible variety of ethical codes. The contrary is the case. Modern societies practice moral parochialism under the mask of promoting univeral ethics. By exposing the essential incongruity between any power-assisted ethical code on the one hand, and the infinitely complex condition of the moral self on the other, and by exposing the falsity of society's pretence to be the ultimate author ... of morality, the post-modern perspective shows the relativity of ethical codes and of the moral practices they recommend or support to be the outcome of the politically promoted parochiality of ethical codes that pretend to be universal, and not of the "uncodified" moral condition and moral conduct which they decried as parochial' (Bauman 1993: 15).

PROXIMITY From what follows it will be understood that the approach to ethics which Bauman describes above owes a great deal of its philosophical underpinnings to Emmanuel Lévinas' approach to ethics *as first philosophy*,[4] with its main motto of 'ethical proximity'.[5] Having made clear what the ethics of proximity entail philosophically, I will then indicate the points of contention between my own and Bauman's post-modern interpretation of Lévinas' approach to ethics. If anything, the thought of Lévinas presents us with a most unusual conception of ethics as based on the radical asymmetry of a responsibility for every other which is *mine* even before my freedom.[6] With this, we are also brought to a new understanding of subjectivity and a reformulation of the traditional problem of individuation. For Lévinas, 'my own' ineradicable ethical responsibility becomes the only valid *principium individuationis*. When Lévinas writes, 'Being is - at least in the first instance – exteriority' (TaI: 290), he means that being is caught, and is 'hostage', in ethical proximity. In this connection, perhaps the greatest contribution of Lévinas to modern thought is that he tackled with great success the problem of *egoism*, one of the most difficult notions in ethics and, according to Lévinas, a central difficulty in philosophy since Plato, only exacerbated later by Thomas Hobbes.[7] Lévinas can tackle the problem

---

[4]In arguing that morality 'is not a branch of philosophy but *first* philosophy', Lévinas points to the 'primacy of the ethical, that is, of the relationship of man to man - signification, teaching, justice - a primacy of an irreducible structure upon which all other structures rest' (TaI: 79).

[5]Of the numerous books and essays written by or on Lévinas, the following stand out for succinctness and clarity and are useful for introductory purposes. By Lévinas (in English): EaI, OS, TO (see list of abbreviation of titles of Lévinas' works in the Bibliography). For collections of Levinas' work in English see Critchley and Bernasconi eds. 1991, Peperzak 1993, Peperzak ed. 1995, Peperzak, Critchley and Bernasconi eds. 1996. More recently (1997) a volume by Alain Finkielkraut has appeared in English: *The Wisdom of Love*.

[6]Lévinas steers clear from the notion of 'reciprocity' since it implies that humans are interchangeable, so that one can substitute one person for another, trade off rights for goods, making exploitation or worse justifiable (TaI: 298).

[7]Patricia H. Werhane explains that egoism 'takes at least four forms. First ... psychological egoism makes the universal descriptive claim that each of us is always motivated by our own self-interests such as that I am both subject and object of my interests. A second less stringent form of egocentricism claims that one is always the subject of and motivated by one's own interests, although the object of those interests may lie ... in helping others, enforcing justice and so on ... Third, ethical egoism contends that one ought, always, to act in one's own self-interest. Fourth, the rational egoist, agreeing with the egocentric contention that all one's interests are *of* the self, argues that minimally it is always wrong to harm oneself. Crude forms of psychological and ethical egoism have been successfully attacked, since the positions in question cannot hold as universal claims. It simply is not true that one is always the object of one's own interests, and the statement that one always ought to act in one's own interests is contradictory. The third view, that I am always the subject of *my* interests whether or not the object is myself seems to be a truism from which

radically because he begins with 'face-to-face', or the 'confrontation' between self
and other (OB: 18-19). As Patricia Werhane observes, this 'confrontation' is both
descriptive *and* normative, 'and who one is and how justice is defined become
realised only in this confrontation' (Werhane in Peperzak ed. 1995: 62). Exposure
to the other is 'both constitutive of human experience and the ground of
experience, constitutive of language which is integral to that exposure and its
ground as well' (ibid. 63). The face-to-face is both irreducible and linguistic, since
'Saying' - *Dire*, more literally translated as 'To Say' - is communication, to be
sure, but is not identical to traffic of information. Rather 'to speak' is to make
oneself available to the other, to say 'here I am', as condition for all
communication (OB: 48). Patricia Werhane summarises:

> What Lévinas has done is to provide a descriptive analysis of how it is we find
> ourselves in the world and in a community constructed by the conventions of
> symbols and language, *and* in a world of others each of whom is not merely
> exhaustively descriptive but is in some sense transcendent or irreducible as well as
> of how we find ourselves as interiority (Werhane in Peperzak, ed. 1995: 63).

In this thesis I promote Emmanuel Lévinas' notion of 'ethical proximity' as an
idea that theory, and in particular legal theory, cannot afford to overlook. It points
us (obsessively) to, but also informs us that we are already in pursuit of, an idea of
proximity and subjectivity without which there can be no transcendental identity
of moral subjectivity but only - as in the present day - transcendental *loss* of
identity.[8] This, therefore, is a particularly post-modern thesis, but it is one which
insists (reassuringly) that there is a transcendental meaning to subjectivity which
is other than what post modernism calls subjectivity's 'radical situation'. There is
transcendence of subjectivity in dis-situation. With the help of Lévinas one can
therefore insist that it *is* possible for the subject to be unique among plural others -
yet only through the rupture of self-contiguity and self-identity, when it is 'outside
itself', by finding itself caught in duties not 'with' but 'for' its neighbour. In
emulation of Lévinas I too start my thesis with the primacy of the 'face-to-face' as
the 'Saying' (*Dire*) phenomenon of 'primary sociality' (TaI: 304). Hence,
Lévinas' thought enables me to avoid the justificatory problems of constructing a
community out of an egocentric perspective, or alternatively, an ego out of a
conventionalist or social point of view. Moreover, Lévinas allows us to re-

---

it follows that I ought to not harm myself. But these conclusions leave us in an egocentric
loop from which it is difficult or perhaps impossible to escape. If all interests originate and
ultimately derive from oneself, philosophy, and thus epistemology and moral philosophy,
too, are to be grounded from and in an egocentric position' (Werhane in Peperzak ed.
1995: 60).
[8] A brilliant book on the matter of loss of transcendental identity is E. Cadava *et al.*, eds.
1991, *Who Comes After the Subject?*.

conceptualise 'social relations' beyond the division of 'private-public', or 'material-abstract' since he shows that:

> Social relations do not simply present us with a superior empirical matter ... They are the *original* deployment of the relationship that is no longer open to the gaze that would encompass its terms, but is *accomplished* from me to the Other in the face to face (TaI: 290).

But what exactly are the terms of this 'accomplishment' and 'original deployment'? Let me go back, briefly, to Bauman and review his post-modern approach to ethics. First, I accept his second point that 'moral phenomena are inherently "non-rational" ', albeit only as it is qualified in the fifth point: 'From the perspective of the "rational order", morality is and is bound to remain irrational.' Secondly, in connection with Bauman's first point, I agree that humans are neither 'essentially good' nor 'essentially bad', but I disagree with the inference he makes that this means that humans are 'morally ambivalent'. The universal truth that can and needs to be stated is, instead, that humans cannot just be reduced to an 'essential *activity*' (Bauman 1993: 10-15). In any case, the presumption of 'essence' implies a being which is both existentially isolated (it can exchange everything 'about' its essential existence but not its own existence - since it cannot die in the place of another) and only as 'sociable' as the engagement with other humans is necessary for its own survival. The ego is thus understood as persistence in self-presentation which occurs in the form of self-occupation and self-care, but also in progressively interested engagement with other, similarly self-minded, social partners. Being, in short, is described as if it were 'outside' the control of ethical proximity and obsessive responsibility - as sole self-preoccupation and persistence in being-itself.

Being *qua esse* or essence is presented as being-for-itself which either cannot enter 'fully' into sociality (and must remain, as it were, in a relationship of 'exile' from it); or which enters society but only as 'empty referent' and lack of self-identity, a *tabula rasa*, a living body on which others write their laws. Bauman's fourth point, that morality is 'incurably aporetic', is also relevant. Although I concede that the moral self moves, feels and acts in 'the *context* of ambivalence and is shot through with uncertainty', I want to shift emphasis away from the 'fact' that in Bauman's words '... the majority of moral choices are made between contradictory impulses' (op. cit. 10-15). The ways in which people affect and are responsible for each other morally are fully expressed neither in the *fait accompli* of their actual moral 'choices' nor in the resolution of moral 'dilemmas' which imply (as the word 'majority' suggests) that the individual's 'moral impulses', as Bauman calls them, are ultimately additive phenomena rather than unique, utterly singular and incomparable personal and inter-personal events. In this connection it is submitted that proximity is 'accomplished' in the unique event of *subjection* by each singular 'me' to the universal moral obligation to 'be-*for*-the-other' - that is, to approach every other human, obsessively, as 'the one' for *me* and *my* responsibility. In other words, I agree with Bauman's designating of moral acts as 'impulses' provided that this word does not allude to the innocence of 'spontaneity', but rather denotes absence of personal responsibility. Moreover, while I agree with Bauman's view that 'virtually every moral impulse, if acted upon in full, leads to immoral consequences', I understand this to mean strictly no more than, that the meaning of each moral impulse (its why and how) is not universalisable. Nevertheless, I presume that the moral *obligation* to 'accomplish' the face-to-face though an *obsessive* approach remains of universal significance. While it is true that 'the impulse to care for the other leads to annihilation of the autonomy of the other, to domination and oppression', this is not so when it is 'taken to an extreme' as Bauman says (can there be a limit to the impulse to care?), but only, I argue, in circumstances where individuated morality is linked to irresponsibility, and when an imposed 'economy'[9] of compassion' weighs down upon the individual's moral freedom, creating an artificial divide between its obligation to show compassion to and its duty to respect the others with which it comes into proximity. I am suggesting the possibility that proximity itself is accomplished through individuated acts of compassion. These are spontaneous only in the limited sense of 'not-willed' or 'not intended'; otherwise, their author remains responsible for such one-way actions. I shall make this point in this thesis on various occasions while looking specifically at relationships between carers and the ill, which I show to be based on 'obsessive approach' of the other-as-unique ('unique' independently of, not in spite of, the absurdity of one's health circumstances) in the form, not of empathy with, but of 'substitution' of the one for the other who suffers 'passively' and 'absurdly' (despite oneself), through 'insatiable but disinterested compassion'.

Two more points must be stressed regarding ethical proximity. First, that Lévinas does not classify 'face-to-face' relationship as it is ordinarily conceived of - that is, as a relation based on 'inoffensive' knowledge or 'aggressive' want. The 'face-to-face' is defined rather as *exposure* or *confrontation*, that is, as neither 'stalemate' nor 'war', and as a relationship, moreover, that is neither reciprocal nor utilitarian. Lévinas is critical of the notion of reciprocity because it implies that humans are interchangeable, that one may substitute one person for another, trade off rights for goods, making exploitation or worse justifiable (TaI: 298). In the words of a commentator, the exposure 'reflects on oneself as self, but the Other remains Other; she does not become absorbed in the self but remains irreducible to her usefulness and transcendent to reciprocal exchanges or duties

---

[9] 'In prevailing interpretations human praxis is caught in a net of needs, desires, values, the rational use of means towards chosen ends, exchanges on the basis of calculated equivalence: that is an *economy*. The law (*nomos*) of the house (*oikos*), the law of being at home in the world, is constituted by a combination of natural needs and rational choices' (Peperzak A.T. in Peperzak A.T.ed. 1995: 187).

that are sometimes defined as part or necessary to human moral interactions' (Werhane in Peperzak, ed. 1995: 64).

Moreover, as we saw above, Lévinas' term 'face-to-face' has not just a descriptive use (which for that matter is limited, since there can be no perfect description or 'said' of the 'Saying' phenomenon of human proximity), but also, and more importantly, it carries normative force. The description of ethical proximity, therefore, does not so much 'reveal' the content of ethical proximity as it commands us to be 'open' to the eventuality of a revelation: that our notions of reciprocity and exchange, according to which 'all' social relationships can ultimately be subsumed under 'the same' categories, paradoxically presuppose, as their *condition*, the extraordinariness and irreducibly astonishing character of singular 'confrontation' between self and other. Lévinas can argue that the face-to-face is irreducibly astonishing because of the way he thinks of affectivity and intentionality. The first, most basic, point to be made is that for him there is an affectivity that is *non-intentional*. 'Non-intentional' in Lévinas has a double meaning.[10] It means both 'not on purpose', 'not willed' or 'not desired' (i.e. without an object and objective, aimlessly or gratuitously and 'for nothing'), and also, otherwise than how phenomenology means 'intentionally', i.e. 'of consciousness' or 'existing as an object of consciousness' without prejudice as to one kind of consciousness over any other. Thus in phenomenology one can speak of feelings and moods as 'affective intentionalities', i.e. as variant ways of being conscious, just as one can speak of ideas, concepts, judgements as 'cognitional intentionalities', or of decisions as 'volitional intentionalities'. All these are equivalent ways of being conscious, and pre-conditions for will and desire. Now, since to speak of intentionality (even of an 'affective' intentionality) is to speak of meaning - 'To intend is to mean. To intend affectively is to mean *through* feeling' (Peperzak, ed. 1995: 108) - it follows that the 'non-intentional subjectivity' that Lévinas abstracts exists in the exposure of the self to something, someone, who is more significant *to me* than a source of meaning for me. To enter proximity is, therefore, to 'risk oneself' in the possibility of no meaning and non-response.

In sum, when Lévinas - and this thesis - suggest that proximity is 'affectivity-beyond-intentionality', this means a being affected beyond capacity for cognition or/and volition, and capacity to 'mean through feeling'. The 'basis' of responsibility and of proximity is, therefore, found in the gratuitous expenditure of emotion by the self for no purpose but for the sake of the other-as-other. This is shown in the relationship of self with the 'death of the other human'. To be sure, there is always the possibility of the survivor responding by means of cognitive and volitional intentionality - after all funeral parlours make excellent salons; and there is, further, 'affective intentionality' before the event of destruction of being.

---

[10]For more on this point see André Tallon's 'Nonintentional Affectivity, Affective Intentionality, and the Ethical in Lévinas's Philosophy' in Peperzak ed. 1995, 106-121.

In either case, the process of mourning conceals that the survivor is also affected beyond intentionality by the other's death, in shedding tears to no avail but perhaps merely as a means of 'marking the spot under the sun' where the recently deceased might stand. Unable to substitute my self for my other in death, I am responsible and guilty before my freedom has been contracted by me, in the unknown. All knowledge, including of course knowledge of the other human, presupposes a 'radically passive' experience of the other as what can neither be a simple 'given' to consciousness nor wholly integrated by consciousness as such. That is to say, the most primordial datum in human experience is the encounter of the self with the other human being whose face expresses a uniqueness so absolute, and an otherness so infinite, that it cannot be thought of as merely an individual human being which 'like all others' is threatened by finitude and death. This 'otherness' of each of my many 'others', which does not correspond with any conscious knowledge or affective intention *must*, nevertheless, be addressed in the form of non-intentional responsibility, obsessive approximation of the other and utterly disinterested 'assumption of care'. Therefore, the command to be-for-each-other is universal although it is 'received' by each addressee in an 'obsessive' way, i.e. as if individually addressed to him or her alone.

ETHICAL PROXIMITY AND LAW The thought of Lévinas has already drawn much attention from scholarship, not least from that of legal theory.[11] This is not surprising, since legal, philosophical and ethical discourses often coincide in thematology: as with 'responsibility', 'proximity', 'intentionality', to name but a few instances. I submit, however, that in a theoretical environment which is still, to a degree, polarised between 'individualists' and 'communitarians' we are in danger of failing to draw all the implications of Lévinas' thought for law, politics and society unless we have an understanding of how *exactly* Lévinas uses the terms mentioned above to convey a quite unique sense of how political society (based on co-ordination of conflicting interests, or: the 'order of inter-*esse*') is 'born to' and 'checked by' the ethical face-to-face relationship between one human and the other, not as fellow-members of the human species nor as fellow-citizens, but as the 'anyone', the one usually passed-by with indifference, whom, however, I must obsessively assume to be *the one* for *me* and *my responsibility*, since even in indifference there is bad conscience and guilt. Does Lévinas isolate and privilege affective, non-reflective proximity to the exclusion of the reason, law and justice which sustain 'the social' and moderate its conflicts? The answer, in short, is no. Lévinas does not privilege 'face-to-face' proximity, although he does claim it, time and time again, to be *irreducible* to the principles and rules of

---

[11]Indicative authors of diatribes on Lévinas' ethics and matters of legal and jurisprudential interest include: C. Douzinas, R. Warrington and S. MacVeigh, eds. 1991, D. Cornell, M. Rosenfeld and D. Gray Carlson, eds. 1992, S. Critchley 1992, espec. chap. 5, C. Douzinas and R. Warrington, eds. 1994, G. Rose 1996, chaps. 1 and 6.

institutions (political, juridical, economic, religious and scientific) which govern society. In this connection Peperzak, Critchley and Bernasconi observe in their introduction to Lévinas' *Peace and Proximity* that the relation between ethics and politics is 'far from a blind spot in Lévinas's work' (1996: 160). Specifically:

> In each of his two major works ... Lévinas endeavours to build a bridge from ethics, conceived as the non-totalizable relation with the other human, to politics, understood as the relation with the third party [*le tiers*], that is, to all the others that make up society .... [He] does not want to reject the order of political rationality and its consequent claims to universality and justice; rather he wants to criticise the belief that only political rationality can answer political problems and to show how the order of the state rests upon the irreducible ethical responsibility of the face-to-face relation. Lévinas' disruption of totalising politics permits the deduction of an ethical structure irreducible to totality, the face-to-face, proximity, peace and love (ibid.).

Lévinas, therefore, realises that 'justice' requires calculation and intentionality in response to plurality. To be sure, to 'judge' the other is already to thematise and objectify him. It is to be at least partially 'indifferent' to him, to 'moderate his privilege' of obsessing me as 'unique', for the sake of comparison with a 'third other'. He says:

> How does it happen that there is something referred to as justice? I respond that a condition for the passing of laws and the founding of justice is the fact of the multiplicity of humans, the presence of the third next to my-other ... Do I know what my proximate is in relation to other people? Do I know if the third sees eye to eye with my other or his victim? Who is my other? In consequence *I need* to weigh things, to think, to judge, comparing the incomparable. The interpersonal relationship that I establish with [the other as] my other, must also be established with the other people. There is, therefore, a necessity to moderate the privilege of my other; hence, there is justice (EaI: 84; my emphasis).

Knowledge and comparison, then are *my* needs, at least, in so far as they are analysed in terms of intentionality.[12] Although the 'multiplicity of humans' and the 'presence of the third' are necessary common conditions for the emergence

---

[12]In this connection, it is noteworthy that, against the Enlightenment's claim that knowledge is corrupted by interest and can only truly be knowledge if it is 'objective', Lévinas argues that all knowledge is interested; and that desire, in his technical sense of the term as desire for the Infinite, for the other, is a 'higher form of interest' than is need, since this 'desire for the non-desirable ... is the subjectivity and uniqueness of the subject [OB: 123]'; finally, for him all forms of knowledge rooted in 'need', and analysed in terms of intentionality, are not fully rational but need to be shown to be in relation to the 'wisdom of love' that accompanies the ethical relation. The 'object' of this process is the 'stranger in the neighbour' (OB: 123).

of the 'social' phenomenon of justice, they are not, however, sufficient to sustain it. In this regard Lévinas asserts that although the theory and practice of justice begin by exposing the face-to-face to thematisation and comparison, they must 'ultimately' show deference to a higher sense of plurality than the one meant by additive 'multiplicity' of interchangeable humans. The theory and practice of justice must address the issue of the non-comparable and the non-intentional affectivity it produces in the judge. The ultimate ethical significance of a judgement is not to be found in the supposedly 'universal' (but, ultimately, absurd) validity of truths and the false authorities it may invoke; nor in the perfection of methods and techniques of discerning particularity and difference. The perpetual conflict of subjectivity and objectivity designates a fate of irreducible tension to the one that has to 'be just'. One can never find an external authority to justify one's judgements nor can responsibility be fully 'assumed' or 'internalised' by the 'autonomous' judge. Personal responsibility for one's decisions and actions exists even in relation to one's freedom. It remains, therefore, in excess of the subject/object divide. It is 'assumed', albeit 'passively', by the judge; the latter, anarchically, does not address 'the third' whose presence makes justice possible, but the judged as the judge's unique responsibility. The ultimate significance of a judgement must be that the judge is 'in the middle of the conflict' but also that:

> Justice is born out of charity. [That, even though] the two can appear strangers when one presents them as successive stages, in reality, they are inseparable and simultaneous, except if one is on a deserted island, without humanity, without third (EN: 125).

It would be a mistake, however, to take 'charity' as at once the 'original purpose' and the 'justifying end' of an otherwise strict justice whose purpose is to impose comparison on the incomparable. 'Charity' must be understood as a diachronic condition for justice; it is understood as the being-for-my-other, i.e. as obsessive love and responsibility for the other whom - even in the most formal situation and even if there is no visual or physical contact - I approach as 'my unique other'. *Ethical proximity* (being-for-my-other) is, therefore, a *condition for* '*justice*' in a dual sense. First, as we saw, it is the fact that one is face-to-face with innumerable others who create the need for comparison and discrimination. In this first, rather schematic sense, proximity as charity and compassion of being for-its-other is thought of as that from which justice must flee, and from which it must be separated. Indeed the 'new-born' Justice grows in the belief of its relevant autonomy from 'mother charity'; but it is bound to find it difficult to disengage from the messy, emotional field of interpersonal relationships, where passions run high and where it is charity and forgiveness rather than reason and calculation that often save the day when love and hate clash. But there is a second, non-chronological sense in which 'charity is inseparable from justice'. The impossibility of justice being realised in actual laws is due to the irreducibility of the individuated passion for responsibility by the judge as ethical subjectivity. Justice is unable to justify itself as a coherent order of principles and rules. Because of the lack of authority and the excess of responsibility, justice is ultimately predicated on the individually passionate approach of the judge to the judged. Yet Lévinas warns of dangers:

> Justice emerges from love. This is not to say that the rigours of justice cannot turn against love understood as responsibility. *Politics, when left to itself, has its own determinism.* Love must always supervise justice (EN: 126; my translation and emphasis).

It is my argument, in this respect, that all 'judgements' (including 'subjective' ones, which I mark here by using the extra the 'e', and 'objective' ones, as for instance the legal, often spelled 'judgments') are, from an ethical point of view, registers of non-intentional affectivity. The tension between subjectivity and objectivity in any judg(e)ment (spelled thus to indicate that it is neither purely subjective nor objective), not least the legal one whose author is all too often eager to divest himself of personal responsibility, must be retained, since it points to the fact that, ultimately, the assumption of personal responsibility for one's judgement and action and their effect upon another is not a sign of freedom in the usual sense (as ability to intend), but an obligation which the subject meets involuntarily yet not in slavish obedience.

To claim personal responsibility for my actions and decisions is not only to present myself as their cause instead of trying to ground them in 'objective reality' - a necessary but not sufficient step towards ethical justification - but also to assume responsibility 'despite myself'; are not the others of my formative past also responsible for my actions and decisions today? Yes, but that is not my concern but theirs. For now, I must say 'here I am' and *donate* my assumption of responsibility to the other I affect with my actions and decisions. I must be responsible for things outside my control. I must be concerned with things I do not understand. Through the donation of self-responsibility, through involuntary charity, even the most formal decision-making process is turned into a chaotic field of anarchy as proximity between the judge's self and each of the beings his or her decisions affect. It is thus, I submit, a condition of proper judg(e)ment that there should be gratuitous assumption of personal responsibility by the judge. But it should be stressed that the idea of transcendent 'ethical proximity', and my linked thesis that all judg(e)ment entails proximity, are not quietist. What is important is to stress that the 'social' (political, economic and legal) criteria for justification of decisions and actions (by means of which the interpersonal is universalised, and the anarchy of particular proximities is reduced through judgment, comparison and common measurements) are a necessary but *not* sufficient step towards justice in a world of plural proximities. 'Society' (commonly held to be the additive total of 'different individuals' - and, in this regard, it makes no difference whether by 'different' one means different genetically or at the other extreme, culturally) is *also* the term for the infinite number of unique *encounters* or events of ethical proximity.

In this connection the pluralistic term 'proximity' is wider than what is commonly meant by 'pluralistic society'. Simultaneously with the recognition of the need for a better 'sociological' understanding of society in the first sense (as being 'with' each other, or in a different context, 'inter-*esse*') Lévinas affirms the universal ethical principle of 'compassion' which governs the *being-for-each-other*. It refers to *all* events of sociality[13] (throughout history and beyond, everywhere), albeit each of these events of being for one's other (each face-to-face) is said to be 'unique' in the sense that it is a condition of the individuated self to want to exhaust the infinite ethical significance of the universal principle to be-for-each-other. Again, this is possible because of the way the universal principle is obeyed: as if it only concerned *me* and my concrete other. Each time and in each encounter with another 'I' must approach him or her as if 'the one' for me, and my responsibility. Thus each 'eachother', irrespective of how fleeting the encounter, and no matter how far apart and how unknown the partners are to eachother, must be assumed unique.

Lévinas warns of two dangers in connection to this 'must'. First, although the 'vocation of compassion' is both unavoidable and absolutely necessary for human society, it ought not to be misunderstood (and later be suppressed) as being a source of irresponsibility. Lévinas not only says that the self is 'hostage to the other' (i.e. bound to be obsessed), but also that obsessive *responsibility* is the *only right 'I' have* before the other to whom otherwise 'I owe everything'. Sociality begins neither in self-assertion nor in passivity as absence of action. It begins in the radical passivity of the self which consists of an ineluctable activity: one could speak of the 'assertion of my right' to be responsible for others rather than just myself - or the right to care. This relation is exemplified by the parent and child. 'Child' means the being who matters to others for more than its 'difference' - since, in so far as it is 'produced' by its parents, its 'difference' is not by itself a source of individuation *vis-à-vis* its genitors and its race; nevertheless, the child is nurtured and cared for 'obsessively' as if 'the only one' of its kind that matters to the parent (see especially the chapter on 'Fecundity' in TaI). 'Radical passivity' as a condition for individuation corresponds to being's engagement in, but not 'belonging to' humanity. There is a kind of interpersonal relation which is full of

---

[13]Lévinas often uses the words 'social' and 'society' interchangeably with 'proximity' and 'face-to-face' to indicate the dual relationship between *autrui* (who demands the dedication of 'my whole soul, heart, all my forces') and me. By contrast I will systematically distinguish between, on the one hand, 'proximity' or 'face-to-face' which indicate dual intersubjective (or interpersonal) relationships, and, on the other, 'social' or 'society' to indicate 'collective' or 'additive' relationships.

alterity and yet is not indifference. It is charity but not exchange, and a condition for *disinterested* enjoyment by the self of the other person's difference.[14] And it is a way of relating *both* to humanity 'in general' and to the other person as unique.[15] Every multiple inter-subjective association is exposed to it in the the plurality and infinity of human ethical proximity, i.e. events of face-to-face encounter governed by the obsession and passion for the other-as-other - that is, by love. But the erotic relation too is from the start 'impregnated' with the idea of responsibility for the third, represented by the idea of a possible child, i.e. of an anarchic visitor who comes to interrupt the complacency and synchronism of the couple.

How is it that Lévinas' 'pre-originary' state of subjective 'radical passivity' is not an entitlement to irresponsibility? There can be no enjoyment of alterity without an act of 'good violence' whereby I assume my other under my care and claim him/her for my responsibility. However, in so far as one refuses one's responsibility for the 'good violence' of one's non-intentional, one-way emotions and acts of compassion (*including*, for Lévinas, the liberal act of recognising each person as holder of 'a-priori' rights irrespective of situation), the being-for-the-other which prompts compassion loses its meaning. The divestment of responsibility for exercising my right to obsessive responsibility and the search for external 'authority' and 'truth' burdens compassion with the *selfish* act of justification to third people - in fact one could even argue that 'justification' is an act of self-care. This introduces relative emotional *indifference* in the relationship with my unique other. I begin to think, 'Am I my brother's keeper?' Thus, indifference can deepen, until I omit altogether to respond to my other's needs, and perhaps deteriorate into what is more commonly thought of as 'violence', that is, manifested aggression and attempts to eliminate the other who perturbs me.

The second danger that Lévinas warns of is related to the erroneous comparison of 'ethical violence' with irresponsibility, which according to this thesis is increasingly realised in the western world. Due to the modern philosophical ideas on freedom and agency it has become impossible to conceive of an act of responsibility that may be 'obsessive', phenomenologically speaking 'non-intentional' and ethically speaking 'radically passive', let alone to accept that such states of being as we describe as 'pure' or 'meaningless' emotion may constitute *the source* of all responsibility. In these circumstances we are in danger

---

[14]Lévinas is referring to the notion of 'disinterest' almost throughout the entirety of his work. Maurice Blanchot describes Lévinas' notion of responsibility in terms of 'a gift, not as the gracious act of a free subject, but as detachment, a disinterestedness which is *suffered* and whereby, beyond all activity and all passivity, patient responsibility endures all the way to 'substitution', 'one for the other'. Thus is the infinite given without being able to be exchanged' (M. Blanchot 1986: 109).

[15]To demonstrate we can look again at the parental relationship. I return to this point later, in n. 63 of Chapter 3.

of overlooking our human *right* (and, according to this thesis, source of all posterior juridically recognised human rights) to *be*, strictly speaking, *for*-each-other without having to have a prior sociological understanding of 'we'. In the modern west, I claim, we have in the last few centuries been irresponsibly indulging our 'liberal pathos' - a passion for the transcendental value of each human being. An apology[16] is often missing today from the exercise of reason: we are together, 'with each other', for no other reason than being-*for*-each-other anarchically and gratuitously - 'for nothing'. The juridical institutions, for instance, on which this thesis focuses, prove from a socio-legal point of view unable to 'translate' into their discourses of universalised morality, and into the codified rules and principles of justice, all that is involved in ethical proximity. Yet, all translation is necessarily a betrayal, and therefore, it is argued here, what is needed, rather, is an apology for this betrayal, no matter how unintentional, in the form of elevating the right to personal responsibility above any reference to authority.

II
The arguments, the theoretical context and
the order of presentation of ideas

Lévinas' views are of value to law. For instance he helps us to understand better the legal principle of autonomy, which is addressing the subject of consciousness and knowledge. Autonomy is necessary in conveying that every individual is unique; however, the 'uniqueness' of my concrete other, as I experience him/her in a certain moment and at a certain place, is more than the idea of his/her 'self-possession' in consciousness and will conveys. Again, my 'proximity' to a unique other denotes my 'affectivity beyond consciousness', and because of this I am more than a subject of consciousness in relation to the idea of the other human as utterly 'other' and - unaccountably - as more 'unique' than 'different'.

In this light, my thesis tackles a series of moral problems evolving around the themes of 'proximity' and law, particularly in the areas of human rights and medical law, making a number of related arguments concerning the relationship between law and politics, on the one hand, and pure suffering on the other.[17] In

---

[16]From the verb $\alpha\pi o-\lambda o\gamma o-\upsilon\mu\alpha\iota$ – to remove myself from *logos* after I have conclusively spoken.

[17] At the moment of reviewing this text for final submission, I became aware of the recent publication by Professor William E. Conklin of *The Phenomenology of Modern Legal Discourse - Applied Legal Philosophy*, Ashgate, Dartmouth 1998. From a quick look it became apparent to me that this publication would substantially have informed this thesis, especially Chapters 3 and 4. Its arrival, albeit too late for the purposes of this thesis, is

Chapter 1, entitled 'What's in a Face?', I juxtapose 'ethical proximity' and the phenomenon of bureaucratic emotional detachment that is the key attribute of modern lawyers and judges (supposedly appliers of 'impersonal law'). In this way several points are made. In the occasion of an 'encounter' between a formal court of law and a comatose man, it is argued that proximity is *not* bound spatio-temporally, nor does it depend on the self-presence of the subject of consciousness, since for Lévinas the subject exists first 'outside itself'. I also show how the assumption of moral responsibility - as primarily a non-intentional or 'obsessive' individual act - consists in approaching the other being as *otherwise than being/non-being*. That is, as neither 'perseverance' in being, having and presenting itself (which is here understood as the 'essence' or *esse*), nor passivity and absence as 'nothingness'. Simultaneously, however, the same type of legal case shows how the institution of modern law fails to express this basic form of *disinterested* being-for-each-other in what Levinas calls 'engagement through disengagement' with the 'otherwise than being'. Since, on the one hand, legal interest is reserved for sanctioning scientific discriminations of 'life' from death, and on the other, law has only indifference for a subject of no interests, that which is retained as 'law' from the various individual responses of the judges in such cases excludes their 'affectivity beyond intentionality'. With this comes irresponsibility for the substance of the decision or action which is to be traced, not to (in this instance judicial) intentional acts and omissions regarding the interpretation of the extant law under which they are expected to subsume each case, but to the act of concealment of their affectivity beyond representation in bad conscience and guilt.

Finally, I also juxtapose certain contemporary arguments regarding the 'life' of the letter of the law. Perennial questions: Is 'law' about timelessness, or about the here and now? And how, if at all, are these two dimensions to law's life reconcilable? Yet a 'fresher' approach to these perennial problems can still be taken. In the matter of legal declarations for withdrawal of life-support from a man without consciousness, the challenge is not to choose between the juridical representation of the patient as holding a right-to-die, or alternatively, as being the subject/object of vital interests which 'perseveres' as 'living thing' without consciousness of exteriority; nor to imagine by means of analogy that law itself is, respectively, a system with a determinism of its own, cutting impatiently through time, or a field of death and inactivity for subjectivity which is then seen as a mere cog. How does consciousness break the loneliness of each being which exists 'with others' in the sense that he or she can exchange everything with them but his or her 'existence'?[18] The emotional state of affectivity described by Lévinas differs

---

most welcome in so far as Prof. Conklin's first premise is that 'modern legal discourse conceals suffering' (at xi).

[18]*How* does the judge's consciousness break the circle of perception with the law he or she reads and the other upon whom the judge acts? For Lévinas, in the event of 'witnessing'

radically from a static state: it is emotion 'for nothing' *qua* deference to death and the 'unknowable'; it is emotion as question which does not contain the elements of the answer; and it is incarnation of *patience* whereby the contemplation of finitude and time gives way to an encounter with infinity as allegiance to the unknowable, beyond fear. Therefore, I argue, to the extent that the institution of law 'expels' or excepts pure emotion from its realm, it does more than 'mask' death. In keeping 'a stiff upper lip', lawyers dealing with issues of life and death also manage to *appropriate the non-sense* of the other's death instead of 'showing allegiance to the unknowable of death'. In sum, if ethics demands that the judging self risks him- or herself in the non-sense of the other human's suffering, legal doctrine on the sanctity of life and the right to die seems to have pre-empted the risk run by judges dealing with liminal cases by allowing, secretly, the enactment of a 'principle of absurdity' and moral indifference to the law. I submit that the question of how to disentangle the legal mind from the temptation to partake in this absurd superiority over non-sense and guilt for the lack of meaning - in other words, how to help the legal mind articulate and claim its 'right-to-obsessive-responsibility'- is greater than the (disputed) limits of interpretative judicial activism.

In Chapter 2, 'Rights as Compassion', I elaborate on Lévinas' point that the modern liberal respect for human rights is not the product of reason and knowledge but of *passion*. With 'rights' we mark each other with an identity of uniqueness. For Lévinas, however, the dedication to the 'universality' of human rights is more the result of a singularly western 'obsession' than possession of truth. Lévinas loves rights *provided* that 'humanity' does not end by meaning a 'totality' of interchangeable, albeit 'individually different' 'rights-holders'. Not: the ego is 'of humanity', but: the ego must be *for* humanity. In this regard Lévinas' understanding of human rights is inseparable from his attributing to the self an 'insatiable' desire for the other's 'individuality', that is, the other is desired as being outside all reference but *me*. Natural characteristics, social placement - neither of these can demarcate my other as unique, as can my responsibility. The world is therefore lived as 'irreducible surprise', and, if understood in the sense above, the evocation of my every other person's primacy and inalienable rights by myself is merely my means of announcing this surprise to third others.

The 'ethical violence' behind our respect for human rights includes the defence of the our right to be surprised by each other.[19] In order that human rights

---

the death of my other the surviving *me* is bound to risk itself in the non-sense of being moved 'excessively' - at least by comparison with what both 'sense' dictates and 'sensibility' allows. But for Lévinas, the most radical effect of witnessing death is not fear or anxiety; rather it is, again, 'affectivity without intentionality'.

[19]Moreover, it is here that I show that what is commonly meant by 'violence' (aggression and attempts to eliminate the other) is understood better after doing away with a certain

do not obscure the ethical violence of proximity, the personal responsibility for the evocation of my other's rights must be shown as *anarchy* and *donation* (rather than be concealed behind the inoffensive notion of compliance with a universal duty).[20] In the light of the above I begin to examine in more detail the ways in which lawyers and judges today employ the language of human rights. Thematically, I remain with reading legal judgements from the so-called area of medical law (this thematology is not coincidental, albeit the reason behind this belongs to later chapters), and examine the evolution of modern law concerning the rights of persons with troubled consciousness, that is, 'incompetent' persons. The American case of *Ms Yetter,* analysed here, startlingly suggests that modern western law is blatantly indifferent to (and has no consciousness of) its provenance in 'disinterested' but 'obsessive' human engagement between self and humanity. The case graphically demonstrates how law takes an interest only in subjectivity which coincides with itself in persisting in essence, i.e. in being-for-itself; and how, thus, the theatre of legal order with subjects of rights as interchangeable *dramatis personae* is superimposed on the non-theatrical obsession of the face-to-face. However, the way out of ontological boredom is not Husserl's 'empathy' or 'appresentation', nor Derrida's 'strange phenomenological symmetry' between 'me and my other whom I know to be an other of others'.

In Chapters 2 and 3 I show more specifically why it is impossible ultimately to suppose any form of adequational and inoffensive relationship between self and other. At the same time, in Chapter 3 I finally reflect openly on and generalise the theme of 'medical law' that I have been investigating thus far. Lévinas' persistent depiction of human suffering as 'absurd', 'useless' and non-thematisable helps to break the solipsism of phenomenological explanations of sociality as a circle of intentionality (between subject-object in perception) and with sociological facts. As such, 'suffering' allows me to reduce being-responsible-for-my-other to being-for-the-other-who-suffers-*absurdly*, therefore, to

---

frustration regarding the nature of acts of 'good violence' or compassion, or parental love which - according to the hypothesis - underlie the invocation of human rights. In short the permanent excess, or surplus of individual responsibility guarantees that the 'approach' of every other human is done 'individually', not in the sense that each response differs substantially, but that in each instance when I evoke my other's 'right' to be I reserve for myself a responsibility which is infinite *vis-à-vis* the word 'duty'.

[20]Each time I have to recognise my other's right to be utterly unique and free; free even from the obligation to be him- or herself i.e. a human being. I owe him or her everything; my own only right is to claim - obsessively - that my other is unique. The danger with imposing an economy on compassion in this anarchy is great in that in 'in-difference' there is only a thin line between the calculated passivity of 'respect' and the spontaneous (thus irresponsible) acts of aggression aiming at destroying the other. Once more the conclusion is that we must re-conceptualise rights 'as compassion' lest we forget how we must be for-each-other and lose ourselves in the complacency of 'being-with-each-other' or the conflicts between the numerous selfish interests of 'being-for-itself'.

beings which confront, and *risk* themselves in the non-sense beyond meaning that oppresses each other. In short, from Chapters 1 to 3 I will have claimed that the 'disinterested engagement through disengagement' which Lévinas supposes as the condition of all meaningful society requires an exposure to the otherwise-than-being/non-being, but also to the otherwise-than-consciousness, or the *otherwise-than-meaning*. And now I argue that the relation of law to the otherwise-than-meaning (which according to my hypothesis commands and governs meaning) is particularly problematic in the area of 'medical law', i.e. the area in which law most explicitly comes in contact with infinite responsibility for absurd human suffering one has not caused.

Medical law could be that area of law where the 'ethics of proximity' could at last be the irrepressible legal ethics. However, if in general today we understand responsibility only as voluntary assumption and duty, it appears that in particular the 'sciences' of positive law and of medicine are altogether 'allergic' to the idea that responsibility exists first and foremost as exposure to *absurdity* and *'for nothing-ness'* (and in this sense, is also, as Zygmunt Bauman would say, beyond the calculative reason of utilitarianism). Setting medical law temporarily aside, Chapter 3 also entails a 'historiographical' journey into the development of medical-academic ideology regarding the aim of, and division of, therapeutic labour in the modern doctor-patient relationship. In this I show how the bad conscience of pre-scientific medicine due to its failures to eradicate human suffering continues to torment modern medicine (which, however, manages to cure more people today than ever before) in the form of a repression of what I claim to be the first call to medicine: compassion and the urge to offer succour. Under these circumstances, scientific medicine is shown to coincide with modern positive law in *excepting* from their respective domains that which I called 'affectivity' induced by exposure to the *absurd* significance of human suffering.

In particular, by examining recent English case law on the enforced sterilisations of mentally ill women I show that when the judge who recognised the right of an incompetent woman to refuse sterilisation failed to surround her compassion with personal responsibility for the horror of mental illness (and instead attempted to found her action in false 'truths'), she laid the ground for even more 'violent irresponsibility', and even the denial of the essence of the right to reproduce in subsequent cases. I claim, more generally, that in the guise of the incompetent woman's 'right to reproduce' we are confronted with the limits of our understanding of the idea that there is a *right to become responsible for* another human (and so to be in constant approach), beyond the constraints set by nature or consciousness, in pursuit of proximity as irreducible surprise. This confirms that 'the other' obsesses the subject of consciousness and language, creating an 'anarchic' 'right' to proximity-*qua*-personal responsibility: a right to say to the other 'here I am for you'. But in this regard, unfortunately, Chapter 3 also testifies to a legal disaster: modern law is applied in ways which not only stifle the surprising character of recognising the other's rights, and conceal the 'good violence' of unique approach and compassion, but also, I argue, worse than exclusion, banish from law's territory the purely emotional dimension of human suffering which is beyond meaning - and so is 'useless' for the purpose of producing an 'objective' - or at least 'subjective' - meaning as 'harm' or 'damage' which could be the basis for adjudication. This is the case whether we look at the English (medicine-biased) 'objectivist' approach to medical law or at the American (patient-centred) approach, irrespective of whether we focus on incompetent or competent patients; and without prejudice to the thematology, in Chapter 3 I examine all major legal principles which apply to the regulation and adjudication of the doctor-patient relationship, and enforce a supposed equality in the division of the treatment decision-making process between patient and doctor. Irrespective of everything, then, 'medical law' has become a little more than the unwanted 'child' of human rights law and criminal laws, and a little less than the (desired) evidence that ethical proximity in the form of compassion for absurd human suffering is a condition for all law. In the place of this evidence we are offered by medical law only the sight of its tragic, and often comical, effort to adjudicate on absurd suffering.

In this connection Chapter 3 shows how medico-legal doctrine is applied in a way that elevates, ideally, either the doctor or the patient to a privileged vantage point on which they stand in indifference to each other - which is also to say, persisting in their differences - and from which they are expected intentionally to 'objectify' the absurdity of the suffering in question and the needed course of action, in an 'objective' or 'subjective' sense respectively. From my point of view this tragi-comic theatre of inter-subjectivity, as it is conceived by modern law's doctor-patient relationship to revolve around the absurd 'object' of suffering, presupposes a relative moral indifference. On the one hand medical law seems intent on bestowing on patients and doctors rights and responsibilities (i.e., in my terms, their 'right' to responsibility or to be-for responsibility); while on the other, the bestowal concerns only 'subjectively' or 'objectively' *meaningful* and *calculable* suffering. This premise must be accepted, given medical law's characteristic of localising and delimiting the being subject to 'absurd' suffering and obsessive responsibility to the so-called 'extreme' forms of suffering which are associated with life-threatening, objectively incurable or/and subjectively intolerable illnesses. It pays to reflect on *why* it is only in such extreme cases that we are prepared to dispel the myths related to the supposed capacity of the doctor or patient to contain him- or herself, even in witnessing the 'scandal' of absurd suffering, by means of their incorrigible, virile 'will'.

From this situation I infer that, if legal adjudication seeks to know society through its pathology, medical litigation is peculiar in that the 'object' around which the conflict happens (pure suffering and the gift of compassion) is in reality a *non-object,* and is therefore legally meaningless. Hence, we can call pure suffering and responsibility medical law's 'useless tools', or its 'objects of indifference'; and in consequence these 'meaningless' forms of being exposed to absurd suffering and responsibility, which are unthinkable and non-quantifiable, become *constitutive exceptions* of medical law. Thus on the one hand, they stand for that which the enforcers of norms relating to the measurement of responsibilities and harm must *not* be concerned with, or must show indifference towards; on the other, the 'suspension' of their significance (they are 'meaningful' only as exceptions to normative meaning) is rendered 'useful' to the contraction of legal meaning, given that one can deduce from their 'exceptional' status a separate sense of 'necessary' responsibility, as opposed to the 'excessive' one that can be shown for suffering one has not caused: there is therefore, the establishment of an *'economy* of compassion'.[21]

This economy has several consequences for medical law's overall conception of the doctor-patient relationship. The latter is thought to sit 'ambiguously' between the principles of justice and of welfare, which are opposed in an artificial divide. For those judges who assume this dilemma, and they are many, the nature of the doctor-patient proximity is at once highly ethical and no more than an attempt to synchronise egoisms: at once 'incompatible' with adjudicative adversarialism and potentially the 'next big source' of litigation. In this light I explain the judicial phenomenon whereby patients are encouraged to seek non-legal remedies for their complaints - although I show the arbitrary delimitation of the contest between doctor and patient about the disputed suffering-related notions 'treatment', 'grave risk', 'health', 'well-being'. For the time being, however, the agents of state justice are reluctant to divest themselves altogether of a role in the area of professional medicine, whose object - as I shall have explained - is now said to be to help being persist in being itself, rather than to 'remove the pains' from the encounter of being with exteriority.

Philosophically, the ambiguous way in which courts now position themselves *vis-à vis* the doctor-patient relationship allows me to argue as follows. If Lévinas is right in pointing out that the common *'vinculum'* between large associations of humans ('being-with' - whereby each human is interchangeable with another) and each instance of individuated sociality ('face-to-face') is the absurdity of human suffering, then this commonality is something that modern medico-legal adjudication conceals. Medical law, in other words, seems incapable of recognising that beyond the contractual and even fiduciary duties which suit the associations of interchangeable beings, there is also the ineluctable obsession with each other's uniquely absurd suffering. Further, whilst modern medical law, if only because of its subject matter, could have become the one area of legal adjudication where the right to personal responsibility (through compassion) would be admitted in order to lessen the false conflict between the compassionate 'impulse' to care for the other's welfare and the duty to do justice and respect the

---

[21]One only has to think of the crucial distinctions in euthanasia law: 'ordinary and extraordinary' treatment, 'action' of killing and 'omission' in 'letting nature take its course', etc.

other's autonomy and rights, the opposite is sadly the case. I propose, moreover, that the exceptionalisation of the doctor-patient relationship in law merely stands for an exceptionalisation of 'ethical proximity' in society in general. It begins in law but has now become the cause of more radical minds. For instance, Carol Gilligan's 'ethics of care' celebrates the (supposed) incongruity between care and justice and, equating 'justice' with adjudication, proclaim certain 'affiliative' relationships to be incompatible with the 'justice model of ethics'. This goes against Lévinas' thesis that 'justice is born to charity' and that the two are 'inseparable', unless 'affiliation' is understood as obsessive approach. In a very different context, Boyd-White's 'legal imagination' focuses on the medico-legal judgment as, more or less, a 'confession' of the judge. But again, this assumes the superiority of the subject of consciousness which is in 'dialogue-with-itself', and underestimates the effect of the self's exposure to the event of its other's utterly unjustifiable absurd and always extreme risks and dangers. Finally, I examine the current ideological blend which characterises the most liberal interpretations of the medico-legal doctrine of 'informed consent' to medical treatment. My aim is to challenge the view of many analytical moral philosophers who presume the possibility of, and then proceed to justify, an egalitarian division of therapeutic labour between doctor and patient.

'Informed consent' by patients also provides the focal point of Chapter 4, in the instance of a case of a person who was paralysed following medical treatment. First, through a close reading of the leading English case on this matter, I show the structural difficulty with articulating legal principles and norms that would *not* stifle the surprise and anarchy of inter-subjectivity as being hostage to each-other's suffering, i.e. subject to non-interchangeable and infinite responsibility. Is it really feasible that one day perhaps legislators and citizens could 'sincerely' attest that 'ethical proximity' is a condition for any 'law' worthy of the name? I claim that it is a feature of all law not only to obscure, but also to proscribe and even foreclose affectivity-beyond-intentionality amongst its subjects (who are legally conceived only 'after' they have contracted intentionality). Further, if 'law' is believed by some to have a 'self-generated' normative and prescriptive power, this is possible only because of the above-mentioned constitutive 'banishment' of reflection upon affectivity-beyond-intentionality. In other words, when 'justice' is thought to be separate from the emotional state of being-for-each-other, then, in this abstract sense, we can talk of laws and politics with a 'determinism of their own'. From the point of view of ethics, any abstract and general normative measures and laws which address equally everyone but are *not* received as if concerning someone in particular, will 'lag behind' in comparison to the universal but individually heeded moral command to be-for-the-other, unless each act of obedience and application of law remains an act of non-intentional contracting of infinite and unique - infinitely unique - responsibility for each other as the one *for me* and *my* responsibility. Secondly, and still in reflection upon the case of the paralysed patient, I begin a distinctive part of my thesis. What is the exact relation between what Lévinas calls ethically transcendent subjectivity (in infinite suffering and responsibility) and today's conditions of loss of transcendental identity? The above case will have shown that although law directs an interest towards a paralysed woman patient as being-for-herself, it only demonstrates indifference towards her passivity. In particular, law of informed consent actually penalised the patient for her failure to be sufficiently persistent in asserting her right to be informed by the doctor. And yet, according to Levinas at least, it is in passivity that transcendence occurs!

In this regard Chapter 4 makes a number of points. With interesting results, the patient figures who will have appeared so far in the thesis (the comatose, the mentally ill, the paralysed) can now be re-thought with the help of Giorgio Agamben's rendition of Foucaultian 'biopolitics'[22] in relation to the Roman institution of *Homo Sacer*. The existence of the latter (a form of being which is considered even lower than that of women and slaves) can, despite its 'marginal' use, Agamben convincingly argues, be seen as 'constitutive' of the western politico-juridical social order. In short, the *zoe* of the material being (its 'raw life' and not yet its political *bios* in which only conscious subjects participate) is 'included' as 'that which must be excluded', or, in my terms, it is included as 'object of moral indifference' and supposed to be incapable of producing affectivity in another. For me, Agamben's argument is original not only in bringing to light the 'exceptional' interest which the *polis* takes in the material sense of the 'living thing' (pure, non-conscious, being-for-itself), but also in highlighting the lapse of disinterested engagement with (and the imposition of indifference towards) the non-sense of the 'nakedness' of human life. This corresponds to an attitude of *moral indifference*. Not only is being engaged in the inter-*esse* 'as if' only virility of presence, but it also appears that the law proscribes affectivity-beyond-intentionality. In both respects, the 'presencing' of the modern autonomous individual, I argue, depends upon the 'exile' from the juridico-political order of the significance of the 'otherwise than being', not as 'exception', but as rule of exception. Can things be otherwise? I argue that the resources for the re-evocation of ethical proximity in the institution of law *do*

---

[22]For Michel Foucault it is a characteristic of modernity that the biological and psychological life of the individual has become 'politicised'. Thus, modernity is characterised by the transformation of politics into 'biopolitics' where the individual counts as simple, living body without consciousness and communication. The living body under constant threat becomes the new location for the exercise of state power. Therefore, from Foucault's biopolitical angle the rapport between vertical and horizontal associations in modernity has also been presented as a problem of 'legitimation' of the exercise of power, mastery, control and so on, but this time in relation to securing the health and vibrance of so-called 'populations' whose mass constitutes the modern 'regulatory object'. I must add that Foucault's 'governmental' interest in the well-being of 'populations' (through attending to individual needs) describes squarely that which Lévinas defines as the order of 'interest'.

exist. In this regard the Greek myth of Orestes-in-exile, who helps to establish the 'first trial' ever in Athens, intervenes in the chapter as prophetic testimony that the continuity of law's territorial empire presupposes, ultimately, the extra-territoriality of the (anarchy inducing) human vocation of compassion and kindness.[23]

Finally, in Chapter 5 I continue the analysis of the 'exceptionalisation' of the being-for-each-other in the western juridico-political order, albeit with a thematic detour. The shifting away from the thematology of previous chapters is necessary, if only in order to show the versatile use to which Lévinas' themes can be put by legal theory. Thus, from the subject of absurd suffering and infinite guilt which fails to impress itself on modern medical law (which is therefore being consigned to the realm of irresponsibility of spontaneity), I turn to the subject of enjoyment - that is, the subject which lives its daily life in constant exchange, as well as the occasional conflict, *with* other beings who 'are' or 'have' what the subject wants. Previously, I have noted the 'exceptionalisation' of the relationship between self and suffering other, and explained how, in law, the responsibility to care disinterestedly for the other's welfare is *wrongly* thought to oppose respect for autonomy. Here, I point to a counter-directional yet related phenomenon. There is an attempt, in the form of the informal justice movement, to 'carve out' from the domain of formal legal justice (this 'domain' is understood, narrowly, as legal adjudication) those conflicts which are said to occur 'naturally' and 'occasionally' between otherwise 'closely related' 'peace-loving' people. The expectations of neighbours, lovers, spouses or colleagues of having their conflicts resolved are said to be secondary to their motive of 'ventilating their anger', hence the effect of the conflict on their 'on-going' relationships and 'functioning' communities will

---

[23]This is not the first time Greek myths have inspired a search to find the principles of Lévinas' ethics inside the Greek *polis*. Let me take Costas Douzinas' extensive work on Lévinas' ethics and law (1991, 1994, 1996), for instance; in particular Douzinas' use of the myth of Antigone as a foundational myth about secular, state law. Antigone, Douzinas says, is a 'fearless and determined' woman (Douzinas 1994: 190), symbolising the subject of unwritten *chthonic* law who defends her sacred right to bury her blood-relative, Polynices, in spite of the legal prohibition by the state. I argue that although this reading may be accurate it is no reason to call Antigone's stance 'ethical'. The ethical event of Polynices' death is not merely conducive to a 'political' lesson. The death of the other human (brother or stranger) is to be understood as the scandalous and absurd disappearance of *my* other into the unknown - an event which affects radically the surviving witnesses, opening them up to the possibility of being in pure emotion for the other who in dying does not respond. Death, mourning and 'burial' - returning the other into earth - cannot be the ultimate events in human relationships. To be sure the anxiety and 'determination' which distinguish Antigone's stance before her brother's death conflict with laws' expectations. But this 'affective intentionality' (this meaning produced by her emotional attachment to chthonic law) is not yet an 'affectivity beyond intentionality'.

be no more than fleeting. In sum, it could be said that if legal bureaucracy has previously given up on love, now informal justice represents love's bitter response: if there is no justice in love and proximity, one may think, mistaking the narrower scope of legal adjudication for the much wider domain of justice, then relationships based on love ought to become 'closed affairs', as if on an island, without 'third' and justice.

In the course of examining the arguments in favour of and against models of 'informal justice' a number of 'side-arguments' are made. Thus, I argue that Lévinas' idea of the 'other' as *my* other makes irrelevant the divide between, on the one hand, the anthropological view of subjectivity, and on the other, the extreme the view that both self and other are 'the same' in being 'socially constructed'. I also show how 'ethical proximity' is irreducible to an ideal form of 'communicative' community (as in Habermas). I further show the difference between, on the one hand, Lévinas' idea of an approach to the other in the form of 'disinterested engagement', and on the other, John Rawls' theory of justice, which requires the subject to put on a 'veil of ignorance'. Finally, I show why Lévinas is not a 'social constructionist'.

Of the two main arguments in Chapter 5, the first reads in the informal justice phenomenon a confirmation that indeed 'Our community is severed. *Homo Politicus* finds its home in the neighbour's loss' (C. E. Scott in Peperzak ed. 1995: 27), and that in our current moral maxims ('legal' or otherwise) in which 'the word neighbour occurs, we have ceased to be surprised by all that is involved in proximity and approach' (OB: 5). The informal justice movement can be read both as an intentional critique of 'formal law' (which is 'justified' by recourse to sociological and anthropological authorities) and as a non-intentional, obsessive delirium, or ethical prophecy. In so far as justifications for informal justice were articulated, I argue, these constituted little more than an ill-theorised, nostalgic recourse to the anthropologist's dream of a 'natural' and 'originary' existence of justice-as-proximity. Under these justifications lies betrayed - because asserted *irresponsibly* as a call to an utopia - the affirmation that justice 'remains justice only in a society where there is no distinction between those close and those far-off, but in which there also remains the impossibility of passing-by the closest', and also that 'justice is impossible without the one that renders it finding himself in proximity' (OB: 158). It is understood that the informal justice movement assumed its right to evoke these two maxims non-intentionally, but also, on an intentional level, misconstrued 'proximity' to be merely spatio-temporal contiguity, and denied that the formal legal adjudicator can be 'the one who renders justice by finding himself in proximity'.

My second argument explains in more detail the event of, and the consequences from the ethical disorientation of the informal justice discourse, from one which aspired to show that 'ethical proximity is a condition of formal law' to one which reduced the singular event of the face-to-face to an instance of 'spatio-temporally contiguity', and which sought to insulate each 'being-for-the-other' from the abstractions and comparisons required by justice and law. For Lévinas there can be no proximity 'without justice' - as required by the presence of the third; in other words, 'justice' prevents the human being-for-each-other becoming a closure: there is always a 'third' to account to. There are negative consequences from assuming the possibility of closure of enjoyment between people without regard for those excluded - to which I attribute the ethical disorientation of the informal justice discourse. Without exposure to the 'third' person (for whom justice exists, according to Lévinas), the 'natural' proximity which its advocates dreamt of recovering (as peace and exchange, with 'occasional' conflicts that law helps to contain) is not proximity at all! It refers to the individual as impatient-being-for-itself, immersed in its own needs and responsibilites, which are dealt to him absurdly but in which he also 'deals' in the market place. Such kind of being, I argue, is ultimately solitary and 'without time for the other'. In other words, informal justice addresses the individual being only as member of the inter-*esse* albeit on a different level than that of law and of its adjudication, which involve extreme (and often unjustifiable) abstractions from everyday 'real life' exigencies, in the spatial or/and temporal sense. In its justificatory part, the informal justice discourse shares with formal law an inability to express that 'proximity' occurs neither in the interminable, 'legal', time of public life, nor in the time of private, intimate life with its relevant impatience, spontaneity and lack of reflection. It fails to show that justice *as* proximity exists in the extreme patience to which the ego is called. On the one hand, the ego comes to exist for its other as unique other and not as member of a group, in disinterested engagement. This ego is obsessed with each 'other' as if unique and as if proximate irrespective of how far-off or how close-by the other is found. On the other hand, this lack of reflexivity must be compensated for by considering the relation of this unique other to all other 'others', as a requirement of justice. The demand from ethics that obsesses the ego, and the requirement from justice that informs it, cannot be separated as if they were consecutive stages - nor can the tension between them be said to be a matter for reflection and work by the conscious ego. Instead their inexhaustible tension must be *suffered* by the ego, in responsibility and patience.

From my two main points in Chapter 5 follow two 'conclusive' remarks. Informal justice proves to be as indifferent as formal law to that which in previous chapters is explained as 'otherwise than being/non-being' and 'otherwise than consciousness and persistence in essence'; but it *is* interested in what has later been referred to in this thesis as 'subjectivity-in-exile', in recognition of the 'exceptionalisation' of the otherwise-than-being' in the juridico-political order. That which is excluded, our individual feelings of being-for-each-other and our innumerable daily obsessions with facing each other as unique in the midst of multiplicity, seeks constantly to re-enter our cities; the phenomenon of complementing state justice with informal negotiation and community mediation is an attempt, not so much to 'include' the otherness of proximity in the rendering of justice, as to 'bring into the fold' and under control the affectivity produced in proximity. In this connection, I compare the ethics of alterity with Michel Foucault's ethics which explain the emergence of the informal justice movement as a recurrence of the so-called 'pastoral' system of governance. In this same connection Lévinas 'ties well' with Foucault. What I have explained earlier in this thesis as 'affectivity beyond intentionality', and later called the 'irrepressible' obsession and violent compassion of judgement, is still crucial here. Under the law-sovereignty model for the ordering of society the individual's non-totalisable elements (absurd vulnerability, infinite compassion) are an object of indifference, and ignored as such. Under the 'pastoral' model of informal justice these become objects for 'care for self' and 'pastoral attentiveness', i.e. they cease to be sources of responsibility, but instead are thematised and operate as variations on the major theme of egoism, mediating the subject-'pastor' relationship.

CHAPTER 1

What's in a Face?
Law and the Man without Consciousness

The face is the meaning of the beyond...[B]eyond what man can be or show of himself... (OS: 93-94).

The-one-for-the-other goes to the extent of the-one-being-hostage-of-the-other (OB: 141).

S'il voit son semblable mourir, un vivant ne peut plus subsister que hors de soi (Georges Bataille).

I
The death of my other and the surviving *me*:
non-sense and sensibility

[Before the other's death there is] affectivity without intentionality ... Nevertheless, the emotional state described here differs radically from ... inertia ... Non-intentionality - and nevertheless non-static state ... Emotion as *deference to death*, that is, emotion as question which does not contain the elements of the answer. Question which becomes grafted on this profound rapport with infinity that is time (time as the relation to infinity). Emotional rapport before the other's death. Fear and courage but also, through compassion and solidarity with the other, responsibility for him *in* the unknown (MT: 23; my translation).

In his *Death and Time* Emmanuel Lévinas points out that death, which is experienced only in witnessing my other dying, is irreducibly absurd and un-knowable. Not: 'not known', but an event of total rupture of knowledge before death as an unorthodox 'object', i.e. a non-object, outside the scope of intentionality (MT: 134-5). Dying is not being's passage into a new, eternal life, but its extreme pacification and passivity. However, although death brings about the destruction of being's movements and expressivity it is not to be thought of merely as being's 'annihilation'. The latter view, for Lévinas, only radicalises the metaphysics of presence it wishes to subvert; for it reduces the significance of death to negative being and 'nothingness'. This implies an equality of terms between being/non-being which, for Lévinas, does not become the 'scandalous' and 'unjustifiable' event that is the death of my other. Further, it implies a totality of Being in which mortal beings participate perpetually, without exit, without transcendence. In such models death and birth constitute two radical events *in Being* to which each being must 'attach itself', and make them 'its own', time after time, in the eternal recurrence of human fate. But, for Lévinas, the ultimate event in Being is not death (or the being 'for death') but society *qua* solidarity and compassion between mortal beings. In the concretness of the *absurd* event of the death of my other, 'mortality' does not signify as information of a generic fate; it is an individuated, incomparable event of 'injustice', and therefore, for the survivor, a permanently shocking scandal which calls for sociality even when no response is coming from the other. Nor is the event of death to be thought of as 'a point in time' which allows recurrence and repetition. Thus for Lévinas the event of death constitutes the *durée* of time in which *time reverts to patience*.

The irreducible relation of subjectivity is not the rapport with itself nor the 'authentic conscience' of the being before death, or *for* death. Responsibility as emotion for my neighbour's death is not confinable inwardly by the subject of consciousness, in the knowledge of its own mortality and in anxiety; rather it is emotion which, like tears, spills *outside the self*. Nor is responsibility for my other's unjust death reducible to participating in the ritual social act of mourning, which attempts to fill the void opened by the other's disappearance. Rather it is to be understood as my obligation to be there *for* the perishable other, or '[M]y presence before my other in so far as he absents himself in dying' (MT: 21). All in all, the symmetrical and 'adequational' proposition 'being-non being' fails to attest to the scandalous aspect of the death of the other human for the survivor who witnesses the death of the other human. Death is described neither as a transformation nor as an annihilation, but instead as 'departure' and 'disappearance' of the other human into the unknowable. Death, then, is an individualising force, not in the sense that in witnessing another dying, and becoming anonymous, 'I' become aware of the 'certainty' of my own death - a certainty which supposedly takes precedence over the absurdity of death and allows the creation of meaning. Rather the death of my other, always 'too soon' and 'for nothing', is the event of *non-sense* in relation to which the consciousness of the survivor is emotionally moved, and accedes to permanent 'restlessness'.

Lévinas thus attempts to trace in the relation to death (as departure of the other into the unknowable) an irreducible event of de-measurement in inter-subjectivity which upsets the contraction and consolidation of self-identity by the subject of intentionality. Because my other 'disappears' in death the circle of perception (subject-object-subject) is interrupted. 'I' - as 'survivor' of my other's death - am the unique but not yet self-identified addressee of the universal moral demand to be-*for*-my-other-as-other. This demand is sustained and constantly renewed due to the *impossibility of dying 'in the place' of my other*. This impossibility is the source of my individuation, the limit of interchangeability. To witness death's visitation upon my neighbour is to feel guilt for their 'departure towards the unknowable' ('*Départ vers l'inconnu*'), 'without return' and 'without leaving an address' ('*sans laisser d'addresse*') (MT: 10). The survivor who is unable fully to know or to experience the other's 'death' is thus affected in a more passive way than the idea of 'trauma' conveys. For evidence of this, Lévinas looks at *Phedon* - surprisingly, since this is a classic work on the 'politicised meaning' rather than the absurdity of death. In *Phedon* the task of expressing that which in death goes against meaning and *didache*[1] goes to the marginal figures of Apollodorus and 'the women'. For them, Socrates' death remains in the end 'non-sensical' and politically 'useless' :

> Next to those who find in this death all the reasons to be hopeful, there are also some others (Apollodorus, 'the women') who cry more than one ought, without any measure; it is as if humanity is not subject to measure and there is an excess in death. [Death] is simple passage and departure - and, nevertheless, a source of emotion contrary to all effort of consolation (MT: 20; my translation).

Further, the death of my other affects me even in my identity as a responsible *me*. This denotes an essential rupture in the very notion of a responsible self; 'not just a simple coherence of diverse acts of identification, but an unthinkable responsibility', *my* impeachment before somebody who no longer responds, 'already a culpability - the culpability of the survivor' (ibid. 15). Responsibility beyond meaning and affectivity beyond intentionality is 'my mortality, my death for nothing' (loc. cit.). Shame and the absurd feeling of 'guilt' for not being able to die in my other's place impede my responsibility from becoming crystalized into a certain behaviour. Responsibility amongst mortal beings 'is not a possibility of impossibility but pure rupture ... constitutes this absurdity that renders possible the gratuitousness of my responsibility for the other' (ibid. 135; my translation). In this way, Lévinas posits our relation to Death i.e., both the death of my other and my own death, as a subjection to the *durée* of time, that is, time understood as the patience and diachrony that underlies the intentional psychic efforts of the subject of consciousness to represent, comprehend, remember and anticipate death adequately. Because of death 'I open up to the Different, the without-common-measure, that which no reminiscence or anticipation could [*ne sauraient*] assemble in synchrony' (TM: 24; my translation).

The 'subjectivity' which survives the encounter with the otherwise than being must be conceptualised in terms of pure alterity - that is, in the irreconcilable tension which holds between its active 'intentionality' and its passive 'traumatism'. This tension, in Lévinas, constitutes a dimension of 'height' and 'diachrony' in which the subject can be addressed as 'other'. Before the incredible difference of death, individual difference appears too small to designate individual beings. Thus, individuality rests in uniqueness rather than in difference. The

---

[1] By '*didache*' (Greek: 'teaching') I mean Socrates' 'magisterial' type of speech. Socrates' speech seems bereft of responsibility for the emotional implications of his death for those he leaves behind.

mortal other is to be treated, not as source of information about enjoyment or pain, but, disinterestedly, as *interrogation of consciousness*. It is in its relation to the other's death that consciousness comes to show allegiance to 'the unknowable'.

II
Legal vision and the appropriation of death's absurdity[2]

... law masks death in the sense that the institution of tradition is concerned precisely with the passing-on of structures across and against the blandishments of time. To the extent that law constitutes and transmits traditions as meanings, as persons, things and actions, it establishes the very form of survival as repetition and in a stronger sense as eternal recurrence (Peter Goodrich in Norrie ed. 1993: 121).

In his 'Fate As Seduction: The Other Scene Of Legal Judgement', cited immediately above, Peter Goodrich shows that law's 'masking' of death occurs in the form of the obscurance of time's *durée* and patience by the interminable time of institutional survival. It is not in 'infinity' but in 'eternal recurrence' that the 'letter of the law' survives. Also, the severe and fixed mask of law is put on as an armoury against the scandal of death as a 'source of emotion contrary to all consolation' and 'in excess' of mourning. Further, I argue that as our 'stiff upper lip' towards death, the meaning produced by law also stands for the appropriation of the hold that the non-sensical event of death has on being. Let me show how this happens by looking at the legal representation of patients in 'Persistent Vegetative State' (PVS). When such a patient, whom both the Common lawyer and the lay person often imagine as a 'vegetable-man', is brought before the law (usually in cases where doctors or relatives ask for law's permission to terminate life sustenance), the law always struggles to deal with it as if a still-living subject and/or as already dead and destroyed 'human nature'.[3] For the law, this 'living corpse' retains its essential subjectivity if it can be resuscitated as a subject which either intends to persevere in being, or is already death-like. It is as if the law refuses to be moved by this other-to-consciousness whose existence hesitates between persevering and giving-up. In short, in the law's eyes the PVS patient is of no interest in so far as his/her existence remains indeterminate: he/she becomes

---

[2]For the correlative idea with regard to scientific medical 'visions' of health, see I. Illich 1976, in which he argues that there is a 'cumulative effect of a society in which pain has been medically "expropriated". Pain loses its referential character and generates a meaningless, questionless residual horror'.

[3]The main case-study here is *Airedale NHS Trust v. Bland* [1993] 1 All E.R., Fam.D.CA.& HL concerning the issuing of declarations to a doctor that he may lawfully withdraw life support from his patient Anthony Bland. The extant law the judges considered here was the 'Best Interests Test' developed in *F. v. West Berkshire Health Authority (Mental Health Act Commission Intervening)* [1989] 2 All E.R. 545.

a hastily abandoned body. More generally, this attitude implies a certain legal view of humanity and subjectivity: both are linked to the ability of being to be-for-itself, including being able to assume the alterity of the world under its own intentions and enjoyment; this kind of engagement with subjectivity shows, in Lévinas' terms, a legal interest in being's *esse* or 'essence' - i.e. being's capacity to persevere in the face of all adversity, filling with its presence the 'void' opened by the other. Alternatively, when the subject is confronted with death - where the work of intentionality becomes impossible and subjectivity's essential ability to persevere in being gives way to the anxiety of being *for its own* death - subjectivity supposedly no longer matters to the law: it is a matter of (law's) indifference.

In the USA the problem becomes a right-to-die issue.[4] Decisions on withdrawing life-support systems are meant to respect the patient's past wishes (the so called 'living will'). When there is no 'objective' evidence of such will, a guardian is appointed who is expected to decide 'as the patient would have intended him/her ...'. In fact, this is an expansion of the 'substituted judgment' doctrine which English Common law had originally devised for decisions regarding the administration of an incompetent's property. In the most infamous of decisions made under this law a New York court asked the guardian to reconstruct the will of a comatose patient, even though the court had heard that throughout his conscious life that patient was legally sectioned![5] That the court took an interest in the patient's will *only after* it became inexpressible is an absurdity at the heart of that judgment.[6] This absurd twist also demonstrates that the courts' 'still-life' depiction of PVS patients (whereby life is assembled in a frozen presence, gathered by memory) is also a *'nature-morte'* ('dead-nature'). The actual patient is treated like a corpse: almost *any* will can be attributed to it. In English law, and particularly the *Bland* case on which this essay is focusing, the depiction of the 'still-life' does not raise constitutional issues, but it depends on the patient's so-called 'best interests'.[7] In this arrangement, too, there is

---

[4]The 'right-to-die' for PVS patients had for some time been discussed in the US on the basis of the Common law doctrine of informed consent and of the federal right to privacy. In the authoritative *Cruzan* case the US Supreme Court found that 'this issue is more properly analysed in terms of a Fourteenth Amendment Liberty Interest' (*Cruzan*, 110 S. Ct. at 2851 n. 7).

[5]*Superintendent State School v. Saikewitcz* 73 Mass. 728, 370 NE 2d 417.

[6]R. W.Momeyer observes that where in *Quinlan* the court 'created a legal fiction in having one person exercising the rights of another', in *Saikewicz* the court goes a step further and creates 'a legal fantasy and logical absurdity' in asking the person who undertakes to make the substituted judgement to 'choose what she thinks her ward would choose while remembering that her ward cannot and never could make such choices!' This is 'either meaningless or pernicious' (Momeyer 1989: 157).

[7]In conformity with the he so-called *Bolam* legal principle whereby as a rule a doctor is not negligent if he/she acts in accordance with a practice accepted at the time as proper by a responsible body of medical opinion even though other doctors adopt a different practice.

absurdity. Can the incurably a-conscious be said to 'have' vital interests? No, according to the English courts: it is in fact dead and only 'artificially' kept 'alive'. Yes, according to the *same* courts: as a 'still-life' - that is, a memorable subject of English medical law - the PVS patient is still an English gentleman who dislikes medicinal intrusions into his privacy, and, incidentally, merits a 'dignified' death. As a result, the much more important issue of judicial responsibility for what in effect are 'quality of life' decisions is obscured.[8] It is my argument that the ambiguous legal *co-presentation* of PVS patients as alive and/or dead revolves around one central difficulty of the judges. For PVS patients the end of life has not yet been present. In any case the vagaries of the so-called 'scientific' medical definition of the moment of death as 'whole-brain death' are such that both 'life' and 'death' in such cases remain to be legislated by the judges.[9] In the words of Judge Stevens in the famous American *Cruzan* case, the judges 'engage in an effort to define life's meaning and not to safeguard the patient's life sanctity'. Thus, faced with vegetation, the judges have to assume openly the inventive aspect of interpretation when they 'apply' or 'extend' the extant law. Yet in all three decisions of the authoritative *Bland* case, the judges held that their judgments were substantiated in a simple application of extant law.

In the first instance Judge Brown had unproblematically admitted the applicability of the precedent's 'best interests' test (originally developed to tackle cases of *conscious* patients) by drawing an analogy between the vegetating and the conscious - albeit 'insane' - woman of the precedent. Taking the animal for the vegetable, the self-conscious for the a-conscious, is a liminal case for the powers of legal analogy and metaphor. It appears that such overt animism was absolutely necessary, not only for the willed animation of the vegetable-man as a zoetrope of 'still-life' interests, rights etc., but for the 'life' or possibility of legal metaphor and analogy themselves. The point is that the metaphor 'vegetable-man' would have been juridically unworkable unless it somehow alluded to either of the clear categories: 'dead' man or 'living' man. But A. Bland was not yet juridically or medically dead. Thus, for the jurist he had to be alive in spite of the absence of consciousness. The juridical operability of the metaphor required the repression of what human 'vegetation' is taken to express, namely, a human *neither* dead *nor*

In short the law imposes the duty of care but the standard of care is a matter of medical judgement. Thus a doctor's primary ethical duties are owed to his fellow medical professionals, his obligation to his patient merely being to apply his training and skills with competence and diligence to ensure attainment of the unshakable goal of full health. For commentary see Buchanan 1991 in Pellegrino *et al.*, eds.

[8]For the notion of 'quality of life' see Sen and Nussbaum eds. 1992.

[9]'Consciousness' replaced 'blood circulation' as the 'criterion' for establishing death in the late 1960s following the recommendations of the 'Harvard ad hoc Brain Death Committee'. For evidence of the arbitrariness of the new definition see Peter Singer 1995.

alive but in constitutive transit, whose actuality demands from the judge more than the ambiguous metaphor 'vegetable' suggests.

In sum, the life or possibility of a juridically working visual metaphor for A. Bland already required a compromise of the ethical affect of his indeterminate actuality, i.e. the fact that he was neither alive nor dead, neither essence nor a void. As the case proceeded to the Court of Appeal and the House of Lords the judges continued to apply the 'best interests' test but now with a significant degree of self-admitted contradiction. The judgments continued to take vegetation for a 'still-life' (so that the precedent could still apply), but at the same time, they increasingly portrayed the image of 'vegetable' in blurred and disturbing ways. It could be said that 'still-life' is now also represented as *'nature-morte'*. In a non-fictional or 'non-juridical' sense, the judges indulgently implied, the PVS patient had no interests whatsoever. Thus, Lord Keith observed that for A. Bland 'it must be a matter of complete indifference whether he lives or dies' (*Bland* at 861); Lord Goff found that 'there is in reality no weighing operation to be performed' (at 870); Lord Mustill wondered, 'What other considerations could make it better for him to die now rather than later? None that we can now measure, for of death we know nothing. The distressing truth must be shirked in that the proposed conduct is not in the best interests of Anthony Bland, for he has no interests of any kind' (at 894).

III
The case of common law

...visibility, for the Common law, is a presupposition, not a construction or achievement. It is not simply a question of virtuality. It is always, rather, 'as if' the world is already seen (Timothy Murphy, 'As if: Camera Juridica' in Douzinas *et al.*, eds. 1994: 92).[10]

The face is meaning of the beyond...[B]eyond what man can be or show of himself ... Not sign or symbol of the beyond; the latter allows itself to be neither indicated nor symbolised without falling into the immanence of knowledge ... The meaning

---

[10] I concentrate on vision only to show that indeed 'There is no way to conceptualize the [ethical] encounter ... to think of it - [Lévinas'] "encounter as separation", another rupture of formal logic - requires opposition to the truisms which we believed - which we still cannot not believe ... I could not *speak* of the Other, make of the Other a theme, pronounce the Other as object in the accusative. I can only, I must only speak to the Other; that is I must call him in the vocative, which is not a category, a case of speech, but rather a bursting forth, the very raising up of speech. Categories must be missing for the Other not to be overlooked ... As speech and glance, the face is not in the world, since it opens and exceeds the totality. This is why it marks the limits of all power, of all violence, and the origin of the ethical ...' (Derrida 1978: 95, 103-104; my emphasis).

of the face is not a species whose indication or symbolism would be the genus ...
The face is alone in translating transcendence ... A Transcendence that is
inseparable from the ethical circumstances of the responsibility for the other, in
which the thought of the unequal is thought, which is no longer in the
imperturbable correlation of the noesis and the noema, which is no longer the
thought of the same (OS: 93-94).

How can the 'absurd' legal judgment on PVS patients be read as *expressing*,
rather than appropriating, the excessive absurdity and unjust mystery of the other
human's mortality? Could this be more possible in Common law, which can be
said to uphold the 'immediacy' of the spectacle of the PVS patient without too
much formalism and abstraction? The Common lawyer, we are told, is supposedly
free to view the judged other with 'simulated immediacy'.[11] Timothy Murphy
observes that the Common lawyer lacks a methodology, but instead operates on
the basis of an:

> 'optical prowess' ... [that] sharpened by the inheritance of previous acts of seeing,
> permits an immediacy of vision on each new occasion. This immediacy, to be sure,
> is contained in a certain way by rules governing what can be seen, or how seeing
> can be undertaken, and such rules of evidence can be regarded as in a certain sense
> lessons of experience and/or prudence. But such rules seek to regulate the
> appearance of the world, not the manner of knowing ...The common law ... is geared
> to generating a situation of immediacy, and rules of evidence serve as much as anything
> to exclude the world if the simulation of immediacy is jeopardised (op. cit. 94).

The fact that in English cases on PVS the judges find it pertinent to discuss
the patient in terms of 'vegetable' may thus indicate an 'optical prowess' and a
welcome 'exclusion' of the worldly distinction between the living and the dead
from the judgment on PVS, for the sake of 'simulation of immediacy'. 'The
metaphorical structure thus permits indeterminacy while giving the sense of
determinateness. It permits discontinuity while seeming to preserve the past,' as
Murphy writes (ibid. 90). Here, two questions are posed. First, does the judicially
employed metaphor of 'vegetable' really allow the judges to simulate an
immediacy with the vegetating 'other'? Secondly, does not the very mention of
prowess, or mastery of, simulation already distract from the passivity to which the
other's death points? It is my argument that the metaphor 'vegetating/vegetable'

---

[11]Attention must be paid also to Tim Murphy's more recent book *The Oldest Social
Science*. He argues that the Common law method depends upon an 'adjudicative'
conception of governance that is both 'optical' and increasingly irrelevant. The
adjudicative model endeavours to 'know' society through adjudication, i.e. through its
pathology. It is interesting that this pathological epistemic should prove so uneasy in
relation to the indeterminacy of vegetation; the limit arguably is not to be found in
indeterminacy but in that there is an 'unmeasure' to that which is neither being nor
nothingness (from a suggestion to the author by Professor Peter Goodrich).

is scissile and ambiguous. Let us think of a painting of a cabbage. Do we think of it as 'dead' or still 'alive'? As still-life or as *nature-morte*? The use of this ambiguous metaphor by the judge, therefore, is not a simulation of immediacy with the indeterminate 'neither alive nor dead' of the PVS patient, it is subjectively mediated imitation. One moment the patient is still-life so that the same law can apply. Another, and he is *nature-morte* and the law dies with him. Thus, we still have to ask, what did the judge 'have in mind' - a live, perhaps, or a decaying vegetable? *However*, even to ask this question already implies that being 'must', supposedly, be thought of as closure, as if cleansed from mortality. In turn, 'death' is thought to be life's negative side, its annihilation, a passage to nothingness. In our interest to know the other, therefore, there is both fear of death and a refusal to relate to the mortality expressed in every life-form. In short, there is reluctance to face the other's death in a disinterested way. To do so would mean that he/she is to be faced as neither only alive nor only dead, neither something which is the same, with its life-force, nor a nothingness, when perseverance gives way to passivity. The meaning of being would be searched for otherwise than in essence and closure. The significance of the other's mortality would not be reduced to the survivor's anticipation of his own certain annihilation. The metaphor 'vegetable-man' is not only retaining a comfortable ambiguity in the dialectics of being-non-being - in its scissile nature it already commands a *patience* and passivity before what neither 'is' living essence nor 'is not' dead 'non-essence': it introduces the mortal other as otherwise than being/non-being, that is as Face.

However, I argue, *Bland* was effectively decidable only in the disruption of the dilemma 'new law for the sake of the other or old law for the sake of the same'. Thus, the judged other took precedence before the judgement. Lévinas' fundamental presupposition that there is inexorable uniqueness in the play of sameness/difference is here instructive. 'Uniqueness in difference' lays emphasis on *l'imprévisible* - that which obsesses vision without turning into vision. In *Bland*, the metaphor 'vegetable' did not simply point to judicial consciousness managing to focus on life, or else, being 'faulty', imitating the passivity of death. There is something prior to the 'appresentation' of the vegetating body in the metaphor 'vegetable' as still-life which leads to its apprehension as a species of finite being in general and juridical being in particular.[12] It is as a Face which expressed itself in its exposure to death that the vegetating body was subjecting the judge to an non-shareable and non-transferrable responsibility. The image of 'vegetable' also betrays a non-equivalent relation (a rupture) with what destroys any noema or meaning. The judges were ethically free to engage with the patient *paradoxically* (thus recognising the absurdity which he suffered) by disengaging

---

[12]'Appresentation' is the indirect perceptual presentation of an object mediated through the direct presentation of another, e.g. of the rear through the frontal aspect, or of other minds through their minds. (For more see Husserl 1970 and 1977.)

themselves from his knowledge as 'dead' and his desire as 'persevering'. The proximity which obtains is an encounter as pure rupture with what can be neither properly conceived nor experienced. In it, the judges risk themselves (and the law) in the other's non-sense. Their affectivity is an affectivity 'more passive than a trauma'. Bland's Face commands an *obsession* on the part of the judges which:

> ...runs through consciousness in a counter-current, registering itself as something alien: as imbalance, delirium, dethematization; as an escape from any principle, will, or *arche* produced in the light of consciousness (OB: 159).

I claim that the *Bland* case excludes the 'radical passivity' as *obsession* of the judges towards the concrete *absurdity* of vegetating existence because of its ability as a Common law case, metaphorically to ac*know*ledge (which implies 'knowledge of') the indeterminacy of such a singular existence as well as give it a 'sense'. This is very unfortunate, because it was in the judicial passivity of obsession with a unique yet non-sensical being that I trace the possibility of the judges to decide. As we saw, the decision was legitimated by reference to precedent in a way that suspends Anthony Bland's being between being and not-being. But the vegetable was not 'alive' nor simply 'kept' from dying. He was *neither* alive *nor* dead. He was otherwise than being/non-being. That 'otherwise' could not become the object of choice and the subject of law's interest (essence), but nor could it be brushed aside as meaningless nothingness. The absurdity of the vegetable-man's condition had to be responded to neither 'actively' (in choosing to re-invent the laws so as to prevent them becoming meaningless) nor in passivity-as-absence-of-activity (in mechanically applying rules). Rather, the 'otherwise than being/non-being' had to be responded to in radical passivity whereby the judge lets the law suffer the absurdity of the vegetable-man. And this 'letting the law suffer' is no choice. In this connection, Lords Goff (at 870) and Keith (at 860) unintentionally offer us good material for thought. Both attempted to justify their decision by saying, in short, that if it is not possible to prove that withdrawing life-support is lawful, neither is possible to prove that the continuation of treatment without consent is so. I argue that this admission in effect suffices as a justification of their decision and renders their insistence upon referring to the test of the patient's 'best interests' totally useless. It is a justification primarily addressed to Anthony Bland as a 'uniquely different' subject of law (non-essential, thus exempt from juridical interest, and yet ethically unique), and otherwise than being/not being. And it is expressed with an ingenuity that is at once passive towards the indeterminacy of the vegetable-man and capable of bringing about a new decision. The legal problem which corresponds to the existential dilemma 'to be or not to be' was not resolved but turned on its head: neither one nor the other, but 'to-be-for-the-mortal-other'. It is an ingenuity provided by the conscience of law's agents which surpasses their capacity to interpret the law. All this suggests that indeed:

in universal investiture ... there lies coiled the dispossession of disinterestedness beneath the concreteness of responsibility, of non-indifference, of love. There is responsibility for the unique, shattering the totality: responsibility before the unique that rebels against every category, a significr outside the concept, free, for an instant, from all graspable form in the nakedness of his exposure to death, pure appresentation or expression in his or her supreme precariousness and in the imperative that calls out to me. Behold vision turning back into non-vision, into insinuation of a face, into the refutation of vision within sight's centre, into that of which vision, already assuming a plastic form, is but forgetfulness and re-presentation (OS: 115).

If the impossibility of fully heeding an infinite ethical responsibility points to the possibility of the myth of law as an all-encompassing closure, so the impossibility of this myth coinciding with the real (as demonstrated here by the contradictions of the legal basis of the judgment) points to a possibility of the ethical demand of the concrete other to substantiate the judgement. To trace this impossibility we need to:

... catch sight of an extreme passivity, a passivity that is not assumed, in the relationship with the other, and, paradoxically, in pure saying itself. The act of saying will turn out to have been ... from the start ... the supreme passivity of exposure to another, which is responsibility for the free initiatives of the other. Whence there is an 'inversion' of intentionality which, for its part, always preserves enough 'presence of mind' to assume them. There is an abandonment of the sovereign and active subjectivity, of undeclined self-consciousness, as the subject in the nominative form in an apophansis. And there is in subjectivity's relationship with the other...a quasi-hagiographic style that wishes to be neither the sermon nor the confession of a 'beautiful soul' ... [It is, rather, subjectivity is expressed as] ... bound by an irreducible, unrepresentable past, in a diachrony (OB: 47).

This possibility of the other to give substance to a judgment, or the possibility of the other to speak from *within* the judge, does not require more than the passivity of the latter. If the possibility of law requires the unethical overcoming of the other, read in the judge's final words, ethics would require the 'succumbing' of existing law to the otherness of the other. It would require an opening up of the judge to the vegetable-man in all his affective immediacy, a being stared-at by this obscure thoughtless life that defies taxonomy, an acceptance of the new 'at the blink of an eye',[13] such that it will no longer hinder the vegetable's concrete existence from echoing through and imprinting the judges' subjectivity. This 'radical passivity' or patience, a 'way of enduring infinity, *is* the full heeding of ethical responsibility. It is this passive exposure to an inassumable responsibility that singularises subjectivity or *me* (see MT: 132-3). This non-intentional origin of responsibility before the other, who is always in excess to representation and

---

[13]For the use of this expression see Derrida 1993.

imagination and affects, in excess to the trauma it caused, demands an excessively singular welcome: so much so, that the other falls outside the scope of legal judgment whose intentionality (project) is precisely to objectify a source of responsibility by putting it into perspective, and relativise its uniqueness. From the point of view of ethics and subjectivity, the gradual consolidation of legality of an ethical submission to otherness into a 'judgement' and finally into a 'lawful one' entails the gradual assumption of this primordial non-intentional and infinite responsibility, and finally, its delimitation and habitualisation (its subsumption into the universal and the customary). This transformation of disinterested concern for the other as other into an association with the other as *alter ego* is the communal phenomenon *par excellence*, an active incorporation of the unique and dissimilar into a social body.

In the event, the prior awesome responsibility before the affecting but unimaginable mortal condition of Bland (alive? dead? both?) was curtailed as this other is imagined to be still a living 'patient' of doctors and 'legal subject' of judges. When the doctor responsible for Bland presented him in court in a particular way, the judges grasped the opportunity. For the first, Bland was a 'patient' and the decision over his death fell 'within the normal state of medical affairs' (since when are doctors executioners?). For the second, Bland was thus a more-or-less-normal legal subject with rights and interests on the basis of which 'death could be allowed to intervene' (since when does death need permission?). The extremity of this delirium indicates that the stake is that of maintaining and consolidating the closure of the identity of agent (acting as doctor or judge), of acting legitimately, substituting synchronised competence for infinite responsibility, by sharing the unbearable burden of one's own responsibility that fell on each one, but also upon their egos. Faced with a condition which has affected them individually in a way that cannot be properly thought, law is made possible through their impatience. They animated the precedent law as they animated the lost ego of Bland, a zoetrope of rights and interests just like their own, a still-life which resembles them, and exists for them.

IV
The other as 'living-thing' and legal closure:
'freedom [from the other] or death!'

I submit that for a genuinely critical analysis of such cases we need to negate law's false dilemma which opposes freedom from otherness to death, and insist that in the event of the 'injustice of death', in relation to which exist all injustices, the subject of consciousness is capable of surviving outside itself, albeit with the 'shame' of its inability, due to his limited faculties and sensibility, to 'substitute' itself for the other who dies - a shame which is greater than guilt, and which becomes responsibility rather than inertia. Yet when the critical legal scholar discusses the closure of legal meaning he *equates* judicial inactivity with death (e.g. Peter Goodrich in 'Fate as Seduction' in Norrie, ed. 1993: 116-142).[14] But was the *Bland* case entirely a matter of personal choice? 'Choice' has a meaning so long as the judges saw the vegetable as either alive or dead. But what can we claim to be the *sense* of choice before what is neither merely alive nor merely dead? The judges of the man without consciousness *did* confess (and also lamented) their inevitable subjectivism.[15] Although the court supposedly only decided that the decision of the doctor to withdraw life-support 'has always been lawful - since time immemorial'- and that it is up to the doctors to determine 'objectively' whether such a course of action would be in the patient's 'best interests', this decision 'remains ethical, not medical, and there is no reason in logic why on such a decision the opinion of the doctor should be so decisive' (at 895). But was the (denied) personal responsibility of the judges really governed by their 'secret' intentions/anxiety *vis-à-vis* the dilemma 'to be or not to be', which are 'hidden' in the depths of their psyche? If so, one can forget the particular vegetable-man altogether: he is no more than the 'skull' in the hands of the judge-as-Hamlet. I argue that this view of the problem may be as restrictive as Hamlet's famous dilemma is banal. Finding out what the judge knew and felt about the 'passage' of being into non-being, from essence to nothingness, does not yet answer how the judge is *affected* by the arrested transit of the vegetable-man who is *neither* alive *nor* dead. The latter is not just vegetating in the sense that he is 'between life and death', being and non-being. He is *otherwise-than-being/not-being*. Must we, then, equate the effect that this other has on the judge with the latter's reaction to either being or non-being? If indeed, in the encounter with the vegetable-man, the dialectics of being/non-being is to be transcended, a different premise for ethical analysis is required if we are to understand fully the judicial attitudes to PVS. The vegetable-man incarnates for the survivor the absurd and

---

[14]For a different perspective see Rose 1996.

[15]Judge Hoffman of the Court of Appeal: '... if the judge seeks to develop new law to regulate the new circumstances, the law so laid down will of necessity reflect the judge's views on the underlying ethical questions, questions where there is a legitimate division of opinion' (*Bland* at 879). Lord Brown-Wilkinson says the doctor's decision to either continue or withdraw life-support in this case 'in the best interests of the patient ... may well be influenced by his own attitude to the sanctity of human life' (ibid. at 875). And Lord Mustill: 'If the criteria for the legitimacy of the proposed conduct are essentially factual, a decision upon them is one which the Court is accustomed to perform ... If, however, they contain an element of ethical judgement, for example if the law requires the decision maker to consider whether a certain course is "in the best interests of the patient" [his inverted commas], the skill and experience of the judge will carry him only so far .... When the intellectual part of the task is complete and the decision maker has to choose the factors which he will take into account ... the judge is no better equipped, though no worse, than anyone else. In the end, it is a matter of personal choice dictated by his or her background. Legal expertise gives no special advantage to her' (at 886).

purely unknowable dimension to being's mortality. But it also calls for the substitution of both legal interest and indifference (respectively, towards the other's being/having and not-being/not having) with *radical passivity.*

More problematic than the question of hermeneutics, I submit, is that law's interest in PVS patients is directed to their blind, biological persistence, as if pure 'living thing' or '*vivant*'.[16] This persevering being is entirely blind to, and ignorant of, the external provenance of the substances which sustain it. The oxygen, food or medicine which is pumped into it, is automatically 'assumed' by it. All in all, the vegetating patient (who was fed and sustained only thanks to exterior others) is 'known' and 'desired' by the court as:

> the living thing [*le vivant*] [which] exists in totality as totality, as if it occupied the centre of Being, in being its source ... For it, all the forces which traverse it are always already assumed, [it] experiences these forces as if they were already integrated in its needs and enjoyment. That which the thinking being perceives as exteriority which requires work of appropriation, is experienced by the [thoughtless] living thing as essentially immediate, as both element and *milieu* ... Its senses ... do not bestow on it anything other than sensations. It *is* its sensations. This sensibility [without consciousness] is of a consciousness without thought...without problems, that is, without exteriority ... intimity of being which occupies the centre of its own world ... consciousness without the consciousness to which correspond the terms unconscious and instinct. The interiority which, for the thinking being is opposed to exteriority, is played in the living thing as absence of exteriority. The identity of the living thing ... is essentially the Same, the same which determines the Other, without the Other ever determining the Same. [In so far as the living thing is concerned] if the Other ever affects it - if exteriority touched it - this would kill the instinctive being. The living thing lives under the sign of *freedom* from the other *or death* (Lévinas, MT: 25-6; my translation).

In the ways the PVS patient is constituted juridically we discriminate distinctly the phantasmatic nature of the ideal object of legal judgment, which is no other than the 'autonomous' subject of law: 'free from the other or dead'. The judicial emphasis on the comatose patient's 'rights/interests' demonstrates an interest in his 'essence' as 'still-life'; at the same time, the complete absence of emotion from the judgment indicates an indifference towards the patient, as if he was a 'lost case' or already dead. In *Bland*, the important thing was to connect this case with the one which laid the 'best interests' test, obeying the dictates of legal

---

[16]For different philosophical accounts of 'life' as instinctive functionality of the organism we can compare Hegel's '*Notion*' with Lévinas' '*Vivant*'. For the first, 'life' is a notion which incorporates the (Kantian) logic of 'inner teleology'. It 'is immanent in [the living thing], the purposiveness of the living being is to be grasped as inner; the Notion is in it as determinate Notion, distinct from its externality, and in its distinguishing, pervading the externality and remaining identical with itself. This objectivity of the living being is the organism.' Hegel cited in MT: 85.

positivism which claims 'law' to have a life of its own, and the arrival at a judgment to be almost a mechanical process. It claims, in other words, the closure of legal meaning, which it purports to be contained in the stillness of the letter of the law which is eternally and universally applicable - a universality and timelessness under which all infinity is subsumed. What is repressed is the emotional experience of the others' death as disappearance into the unknowable, and as non-sense *in* which the judges were called upon by ethics to *risk* themselves.

Ethically, the relationship to the man without consciousness must go beyond the one between *ego* and *alter* which is based either on knowledge of, or on mimetic desire for, what the other is/has. For 'knowledge' presupposes an adequacy of correspondence between ego and other which is not available in the relation of the one for the mortal other. And 'desire' articulates the mimetic identification between *ego* and its *alter* as a dual impulse of being and having which, again, does not extend to the gratuitous concern of the one for the other, who, in dying, departs into the unknowable. What was, in *Bland,* the universal investiture of the man-without-consciousness in law as a legal subject? In other words, who (or, what) *is* the Anthony Bland which the judges insisted in 'knowing' as dead and 'desiring' as still-living? The 'object' of knowledge (death) is that which cannot be known by the judges except as negation of Being. The patient's lack of consciousness in this case becomes an excuse for the judges to relate to him as already dead, 'devoid' of interests and rights, a 'nothingness'. Thus one can 'know' what death is: non-essence. On the other hand, the judges' mimetic desire is directed at Anthony Bland as organism which still perseveres. It is the combination of the knowledge with the desire that allowed the judges to formulate, absurdly, that 'it is in the interests of the patients to die although he is devoid of all interests'. A question is raised in this connection. How to qualify law's inability to step outside the realm of relationships based on either possessive desire or inoffensive and unemotional knowledge? Could it be otherwise? Unfortunately:

> The defining feature of legal modernity lies in the attempt to make law self-founding...to seek ...the justification of judgment...within law itself. The science of law was thus predicated upon legal closure. The thesis on the death of law can be approached as a question relating to the decay of legal reason and specifically to the demise of certain forms of speaking or invoking legal judgment. In either case, it is first a matter of death and of what it means for an institution to die. Hermeneutically, it is a paradox in so far as institutions are by definition legal fictions that do not die; institutions such as religion, law or economics...are forms of (social) life and as such they cannot die...In consequence, to speak of the death of law is to appropriate a metaphor...which is contradicted by the classical principle of *lex aeternitas* and the maxim *dignitas [ius] non moritur* (Peter Goodrich in Norrie ed. 1993: 165).

Can we expect the modern judge to admit that the opposition between judicial interest in being, and indifference to non-being, is made redundant by his/her responsibility towards the otherwise-than-being/non-being? Just how much 'virility' of spirit can we expect from the modern judge who is asked to decide on PVS? Can what Lévinas means by 'ethical passivity' of the one-for-the-other - which stems from each other's mortality - be undertaken as a *project* rather than be simply suffered by the subject, for instance the judge in PVS cases? In general terms, the contemporary re-emergence of the debate over ethics and law revolves, essentially, around the following problem posed by hermeneutics. For critical legal theory the judge is always interpreting the law and so is faced with an ethical 'dilemma' - whether to employ this interpretative possibility to the effect of reiterating the universal applicability of the same (dead?) meaning of legal rules, or whether to introduce new meaning by fitting the rules to the particularities of the 'other'. Others continue to deny that this interpretative opportunity exists for the judge. But what has been common to both these claims is the binding of the questioning of the relation between universality and individuation to this disputed *mastery* of judicial activism over the rapport between law and ethics. I submit that the radically passive and obsessive aspect of the legal judgment eludes theories which privilege judicial mastery over the 'dilemma' universality-individuality.

Two contemporary views in which the question of judicial activism becomes paramount for the relation between an ethical demand for individuation and discontinuity, and the legal requirement for universality and continuity, are those of Drucilla Cornell and Stanley Fish.[17] The former, focusing on the 'unavoidable character' of judicial inventiveness, calls for it to be put to 'good use'. She argues that the judge heeds his/her ethical responsibility before the singular individual of the particular case if he/she *acts* so as to 'imaginatively recollect' the relation of this other with law. Through this 'imaginative recollection', the judge puts the individual in a negative perspective to law, and conceives of or imagines him/her beyond the 'traditional exclusions of established law'.[18] Fish maintains that no matter how inventive the judge, he/she is ultimately bound to reinstate the idea of law as having a 'life of its own', if only 'mythically', by linking his/her decision to an (albeit illusive) belief in the full readability of existing law and the intention of the 'founding fathers'. Further, according to legal theory a juridical decision is legally sound, not only if it is substantially in coherence with a system of law, but also if it is 'mythically' so. Evidently in both Cornell's and Fish's positions, the question of the ethical in the judgment is answered with a prejudice in favour of judicial activism. Whether accepted or denied, judicial interpretative activism appears to be the only way a judge heeds his or her ethical responsibility to judge

---

[17]See respectively Cornell 1992 (espec. chaps. 4 and 5), and Fish 1989.

[18]See espec. Cornell's commentary of *Roe v. Wade* (Cornell 1992: 146-154).

a unique individual *as such* and not as a generalised legal subject construed according to a universal legal meaning.

However, as we have seen, when the human without consciousness and persistence of being encounters the law, 'justice' commands *patience* and *passivity* before the otherness of death. As Aeschylus put it in *Niobe,* 'from Death alone Persuasion stands apart'. Both Fish and Cornell - as indeed many other legal theorists recently - are readers of the philosopher Lévinas. However in equating ethical responsibility with judicial activism, they overlook the emphasis Lévinas puts on the passively patient dimension of ethical responsibility (which, for that reason, he calls a 'subjection'). The Self as a 'dialogue of the soul with itself' manages only to a certain degree to contain its other in its imaginative depictions and conceptual representations. But as the Self's presentation requires this correlation, Self is constant strife, and activity towards a project *a priori* never enough. Thus, already to think of oneself as a 'judge' and of a judgement as 'legal' is to be caught in an active - though never sufficient - strife. First, it is to view and comprehend the unique judged *as if an object of judgment* rather than a source of responsibility. Second, it is to view and understand the ethically bound judgment *as if a mechanical function* within law's closed system. The two 'as if's are synchronic aspects of a judicial activity which essentially boils down to the labour of visual and conceptual metaphor. This labour is concomitant with the judge's evasion of his or her personal individuated ethical responsibility. Further, this concomitance is the possibility of a judgment. Nevertheless it is a labour never sufficient, always inconclusive, and thus always susceptible to the ethical responsibility from which it flees.

The most important lesson from the *Bland* case is that the so-called dilemma between individuation and universality is superseded as we come to understand that the 'link' between universality and individuation is not so much a link as a rupture, whereby the former is the 'obsession' of the latter. I argue, moreover, that between individuated justification and universalized legitimation, judicial activism *appears necessarily to side with the latter*. The ability of Anthony Bland's judges to present him metaphorically as a juridically qualified 'life or death' alludes to law's self-representation as 'still-life' and systemic closure of legal meaning. The judges seem to think that, 'yes, there is freedom beyond the boundaries of the law - but, acknowledging this will be law's death'. Cornell's 'interpretative freedom' of the judge should be able to act as the 'consciousness' of the law, capable of shattering law's illusive belief in its autonomy as closure. The judges should be able to admit that the blindness of such a patient's existence to his exteriority, his lack of consciousness that prevents him from feeling for those who feed him, already makes him a dead human, albeit still a human. However, I showed that their interpretative *activity* is inescapably directed towards representing the patient's mechanical, 'blind' existence as full 'life', or else the lack of it as death. Thus, Cornell's and Fish's arguments are valid only for the wrong reasons. In terms of ethics and subjectivity, it would be the judicial inventiveness which Fish seeks to deny or relativise that helps maintain the illusion (as it may be) that the 'still-life' (or *nature-morte*) of the letter of the law is 'threatened' by their being. And conversely, it is in the break or rupture of judicial activity, the suspension even of Cornell's moral-juridical project, that the impact of the ethical demand of a singular 'other' is guaranteed in the judgment.

Peter Goodrich's view that 'death belongs to the biography' of law as an 'active principle of disintegration' of legal judgment suggests an affinity with Heidegger's analytic where death is the imperative that ordains singular existence. Specifically, in Heidegger authenticity is 'achieved' by 'projecting' oneself towards death. Another man's death makes me sure of my own. In this way death becomes intimately personal for the survivor: its 'certainty' singularizes being by provoking it to 'project itself towards its own death', and, in so doing, to acquire its own time. 'The singular essence of an existence is engendered in the assembling not of its parts or its faculties but of its times. For according to the modern analysis, time is the internal order or structure of the soul; time is *principium individuationis*' (A. Lingis 1989: 111). Further, death provides conscience with the modality for a 'purposeful existence'. Heidegger attributes authentic transformation to the sense of mortality and the anxiety produced by the anticipation of my death. Though 'of death we know nothing', anxiety *knows*: conscience anticipates with certainty and thus knows the imminent threat of nothingness that measures its existence. And yet:

> it is not the nothingness that delimits and individuates, for of itself the confrontation with nothingness which has no front lines in anxiety is dissolute and disintegrating and the anticipation of death is already a dying. The apprehension of the existence whose scope and span are measured by nothingness, by death, must be a life's *own work, a work that is positive and internal* ... The anxious conscience anticipates - that is, does not merely represent but projects me into - the full expanse of what is possible for me, anticipates the uttermost limits of the possible, unto the possibility of impossibility, of irreversible and definitive impotence. Once one has anticipated one's death one has anticipated what is possible, all that is possible (Lingis 1989: 111).

If Being by itself 'projects' itself unto it, death, in consequence, should not be thought of as intrinsically unthinkable and unintelligible, but on the contrary, as the 'only certainty', to which Being anxiously clings. The 'deathbound propulsion of our existence is the spirit itself ... is what makes our movements comprehending and our existence exultant, ecstatic - the understanding that is authentic thought' (Lingis 1989: 109). I submit that from Goodrich's 'Heideggerian' view of death as an opportunity for internal 'work' towards an authentic, personalised understanding of death, the decision in *Bland* contains 'inauthentic', anonymous judicial thought. *Bland* would be a 'subordinate or crippled legal judgment' (Goodrich in Norrie 1993: 118); for its authors clearly abdicated their 'competence to speak of the event' which requires the judges to 'disengage' themselves, 'momentarily', from the principles of reproduction of law (ibid. 131). For Goodrich, the judges in *Bland* are ethically responsible for 'squandering' their death-inspired 'ability to move from a field of reproduction, or of law, to a field which is demarcated around the event and which by virtue of its externality shatters the pre-existent sentence or competence' (ibid. 121). The judges, that is, must have failed to 'grasp' that '[D]eath is what passes, what succeeds, unacknowledged from father to son ... which, as an event, cannot be contained ... [but rather] ... makes containment possible ...' (ibid.). Further, the judges in the case of the man-with-no-consciousness must have failed to produce a judgment which addresses death with such figurative or literary means as are appropriate for depicting death to be 'the condition or possibility of sociality ... precisely because it limits and so delimits the subject and in consequence displays the necessity of the social' (ibid.).

There is indeed much value in any view which invites the law to confront death 'authentically', i.e. otherwise than as mere negation of life and as the catastrophic 'end of time'. An authentic judgement would have required the judges to drop out of the interminably 'public', 'natural' and universal and 'objective' time, and in 'judging' the other's death, to acquire a time of their own. In all this, the judgment on the event of Anthony Bland's death must have failed, for:

the practice of judgment, to be just or ethical ... must exceed the terms and constraints of merely positive and municipal rule (ibid.).

I want to conclude by suggesting that Goodrich's views can be radicalised from a Lévinasian perspective. Lévinas would warn against the belief that there are 'appropriate' rhetorics or aesthetics to match the ethical guilt and constant accusation of the other human's disappearance into the unknown. In the instance of *Bland,* for example, it is not so important to decide whether the metaphor 'vegetable' (still ambiguous: still-life or *nature-morte?*) is 'appropriate' or not. Goodrich is right to point out that death is not an 'external force threatening legality' but an 'internal quality' of legal judgment. But he is wrong to assert that the only possible alternative to an authentic approach to the other's death would be - in rhetorical terms and with regard to judgment -

vanitas or decadence and in psychological terms ... an instinct or drive negating both pleasure or reproduction ... [which] ... [P]hilosophically ... would be the death of the soul, of the spirit of law: an extinction which in metaphysical terms is represented as closure or the failure to create, and mundane terms as injustice in the precise sense of *ressentiment,* passivity or existential inauthenticity, namely a being in flight from death (Goodrich in Norrie ed. 1993: 120).

I submit, in this connection, that beyond the authenticity and *vanitas* of being which exists *for* death or 'in flight from' death there is a passivity of being as the otherwise-than-being/non-being. The ultimate individuating act of subjectivity is not to 'make its own' the death of its other (as a confrontation with 'nothingness'); it is rather to risk itself in the other's mortal non-sense. Nor is it to 'use' the other's death 'in order' that its own existence become 'purposeful'; rather it is to witness the scandal of my other dying 'for nothing'. The most significant insight in Lévinas' view on the death-of-the-other-human is that it cannot become entirely of public interest or 'politicised'[19] *because* it calls, not so much for the 'work' by which the survivor appropriates death's absurdity, as for disinterested and patient *deference* towards it. Emotion as deference towards death - that is, emotion as question which does not bear elements of reply; a question which opens our most profound relationship with time as infinity - in patience. To be sure, in this purely emotional rapport with the other's death there is also fear and/or courage, but more importantly, through obsessive compassion and solidarity there is the survivor's responsibility for the death of the other as his or departure into the unknowable. In short for Heidegger individuation results from the appropriation by one being of the absurdity of its other's death since the event wherein another disappears matters only as confirmation of the survivor's own mortality. By contrast in Lévinas the *unicity* of the surviving *me* (i.e., the ethical *subjectum* as guardian of its other which survives the death of this other) requires '*risking*' an attitude of existential *patience* even in the eventuality of non-sense and non-response. In terms of Goodrich's 'Fate as Seduction' it is not clear whether this eventuality of non-sense remains of concern. In any case Lévinas insists that:

> patience *must* be risked in the eventuality of non-sense, patience which is even owed before the discovery [*dé-couvertment*] of arbitrariness - therefore, a non-dischargeable patience is possible. It requires an opening to a dimension which is discovery, ridiculing the nobility of patience ... marring its purity. If patience has a sense in so far as it is inevitable obligation [fate] this meaning becomes sufficient and institutionalised ... unless there remains a *soupçon* of non-sense. The egoicity of me must, therefore, include the risk of non-sense and madness. If the risk is not there, patience would acquire a status, would lose its passivity (MT: 23; my translation).[20]

---

[19] For a different view on the 'biopolitics' of indifference to death see Agamben 1995.

[20]'doit se risquer dans l'éventualité du non-sens, patience qui se doit même devant un découvert de l'arbitraire - alors une patience non acquitable est possible. Il faut une ouverture sur une dimension qui est un découvert, ridiculisant la noblesse ou la pureté de la patience, l'entachant. Si la patience a un sens en tant qu'obligation inévitable, ce sens devient suffisance et institution s'il n'y a pas au-dessous un soupçon de non-sens. Il faut donc qu'il y ait dans l'égoicité du Moi le risque d'un non-sens, d'une folie. Si le risque n'etait pas là, la patience aurait un statut, elle perdrait sa passivité' (ibid. 23).

CHAPTER 2

Rights as Compassion:
Law and the Incompetent

Justice is born out of charity. The two can appear strangers when one presents them as successive stages; in reality, they are inseparable and simultaneous, except if one is on a deserted island, without humanity, without third ... Justice emerges from love. This is not to say that the rigours of justice cannot turn against love understood as responsibility. Politics, when left to itself, has its own determinism. Love must always supervise justice (OB: 125-126).

The rights claimed under the title rights of man, in the rigorous and almost technical sense which that expression has taken on since the eighteenth century - the right to respect for the human dignity of the individual, the rights to life and liberty, and equality before the law for all men - are based on an original sense of the right, or the sense of an original right. And this is the case, independently of the chronology of the causes, the psychological and social processes and the contingent variations of the rise of these rights to the light of thought. They are probably, however complex their application to legal phenomena may be, the measure of all law, and no doubt, of its ethics (OS: 116).

I
Lévinas' disinterested intensities and 'good violence'

It is my premise that in modern liberal societies the use of representations and categories that constitute public memory and common knowledge do not so much express or depict 'real' social categories as create or construct those very things. In so far as law is concerned, this phenomenon can be described as a 'metaleptic' reversal in liberal law, whereby we see abstract identities of meaning - the abstract right to self-determination for example - rather than the unique moral situations that actually give rise to those apparent identities. This phenomenon plagues the language of liberal law. In this connection the philosophy of Lévinas offers us guidance. In his lecture on 'Substitution', language is interpreted, not as reciprocal traffic of information, nor as possessive desire,[1] but as presentation of the one for

---

[1] In this possessive sense 'desire' would be called a 'need' by Lévinas, by contrast to his technical use of the term 'desire' as obsession with infinity. In *Totality and Infinity*, Lévinas' phenomenological critique of the economical attitude entails this fundamental distinction between needs *(besoins)* and ethical desire *(désir)*. Later, in *Otherwise than Being* Lévinas analyses the ontological structure of 'economical existence'. Peperzak sums up: '[Ethical] desire transcends economy ... just as the Good ... is shown to transcend ontology. Desire is

the sake of the other (S, see Bibliography). In language, being says 'here I am'. The ethical desire for proximity with a unique other is irreducible to consciousness and thematisation. It is an insatiable desire for an *anarchic* relationship with a singularity, without the mediation of any principle or ideality. The face-to-face is not identical with the supposedly inoffensive relationship based on knowledge and representation, where everything and everyone is equivalent, and therefore subject to use of metaphor and metalepsis.

Moreover, it is apparent throughout Lévinas' work that his idea of 'justice' is that of peace and non-violence; and moreover, that for him justice is the starting-point in any human relationship understood as one of proximity, i.e. a relationship brought forth by gratuitous love or charity which Lévinas equates with responsibility of the one for the other. It would be a mistake, however, to infer from this that Lévinas' love of peace supersedes his love of anarchic proximity. In his ethics of alterity there is not concern only for inoffensive relationships. On the contrary, proximity deserves its name only in so far as in it the alterity between humans is maintained by means of constant 'confrontation' of self and other. Therefore, Lévinas' justice as non-violence is far from a denial of the possibility that, in the words of Jacques Derrida, we must assume an 'originary violence that is also the possibility of ethics' (Derrida 1967: 184). In this regard, suffice it to quote Lévinas at his most explicit. Already in the beginning of *Otherwise than Being* he claims 'proximity' to be first and foremost *approach* (rather than commitment) (OB: 5). By this, he means that in the 'originary' inter-human relationship, the definitive (irreducible) phenomenon is that of a non-reciprocated act of obsessive approach and self-presentation by each other as unique. It is here that Lévinas' notion of a 'pre-original' but also 'good violence is important.

Large, peaceful human associations of interchangeable beings constantly presuppose, as their possibility, certain one-way acts of 'ethically violent' charity, through which each human approaches its other in pure 'disinterestedness', but also puts itself at its other's service. Through these acts each being claims its other to be unique beyond the difference they manifest, and worthy of infinite love, as if each individual were 'the only human that matters'. Lévinas' bold philosophy might be said to constitute one such act. These acts are pure gifts, pure giving even of oneself. It cannot be over- stressed that the putting of oneself at the other's service is not a sign of slavery or self-sacrifice, because the giving 'self' has not yet contracted sovereignty and, in consequence, can neither lease it nor lose it. For the giving self is not the origin of its gift to its other, and so the gift cannot later return to him or her in the form of thanks or gratitude; rather, the self is the object of a universal demand expressed in the face of the other: 'approach me', 'help me', 'die for me'. The self-giving ego of ethical obligation is, therefore, different from

---

not interested in satisfaction or exchange; it does not assimilate or integrate because it is not oriented towards enrichment or expansion. As desire for the Other, it accords with the surprising strangeness and distance without which there would be no otherness ... [P]roximity [thus] does not diminish but rather intensifies [ethical] desire' (Peperzak ed. 1995: 189).

the self-same ego of the subject of consciousness which later comes to reflect on its obligations. It gives itself, and:

> shows, in its saying to the other *qua* approach ... the very de-positioning or de-situating of the subject, which nonetheless remains an irreplaceable uniqueness, and is thus the subjectivity of the subject (OB: 48).

Even if one accepts the above premises, however, it is difficult to conceptualise the act of donating my 'disinterested servitude' to the other, especially when this is characterised as an *imposition* of a 'good violence' (OB: 43). In this connection, in the context of discussing modern liberal ethics and the western world's concern with human rights, Lévinas points out that proximity *qua* disinterested approach is experienced from within the 'pathos of liberalism' [*le pathétique du liberalisme*] (TaI: 125). This 'pathos' is said to command modern politics and law (albeit in an unacknowledged form) and immediately connects respect for human rights with 'good violence'. Why violence? In showing my respect for my other's unicity (which must be there if 'I' am to be a unique donor of charity) I attribute the idea of *a-priori* right to my other. Thus, I violently 'extract' my other from the 'determining order of nature'; I 'suspend all reference' with regard to my other except from *me* (HS 1987: 176). In both liberal and radical ethics of alterity I am bound to effect a 'violent tearing-loose' of each of my many others from all context in order to direct my disinterested kindness. For this I am to be held responsible although 'I' never chose it. It is thus, through the inescapable violence of 'one-way' desire, that the pathos of liberalism begins. I am subjectively 'free' to 'mark the absolute identity of [my other] person as non-interchangeable, incomparable and unique' (ibid.). This violent spatial 'suspension' of my other from all reference is not by means of 'some form of abstraction' because the uniqueness of the other that I desire is sought in the other as incomprehensible. It is important not to lose sight of the fact that Lévinas uses the word 'freedom' to encounter the other in a unique sense: the encounter with my other is characterised as an irreducible experience of *astonishment* whereby the desire for otherness *pre-empts* my need and my ability to know my other ('for what he or she is/is not') or to be interested by him or her for what he or she is/is not and has/has not. If I am free to mark my other with the identity of uniqueness it is because I am the subject of a desire and surprise.

From then on, Lévinas proceeds to qualify this inevitable or 'good' violence by the ethical subject (a me with no *I*) differently from the voluntary violence with which the (posterior) 'sovereign' subject of self-consciousness chooses to *surround* its love for the unique, other as well as its respect of the other's rights. For instance 'ethical violence' attaches to the self's 'involuntary' eroticism for the other. Thus one comes to claim one's object of admiration as a 'unique' face; he or she is neither 'different' enough to be 'external' to me, nor can be fully internalised. There is 'ethical violence' too in the love of parent for the 'child' he or she both 'has' and 'is'.[2] It is for this reason that the biblical sacrifice of the son was never concluded: the offer of sacrifice by the father who 'is' his son cancels the necessity for sacrifice by the father who 'has' a son. Such is the 'redeemable' violence of the human's desire to approach its other human as unique - that is, as absolute other. As for 'non-ethical' violence, this, typically for Lévinas, begins in irresponsibility for the first kind of violence.[3]

---

[2]Obsessive love for and counter-intentional desire to be responsible for the other being that is the 'child' is not a 'quality' that parents are called to 'make their own'; it is rather a precondition of parenthood which operates prior to and indeed independently of the parents' biological reproductive capability and their mimetic desire or knowledge of reproduction. Nor is parenthood a mere species of the category of love relationships. Rather, parental love stands for the pre-original *sine qua non* of all love. As the aimless caressing of the beloved indicates, 'love' is not only an intentional focus or an empathic apperception 'aiming' at another as object which can be unavailable or be lost. In caressing one's beloved partner - even in craving to caress - one encounters the incomparable other, who lies outside the lovers' past and present, in a future 'not yet'. Hence, love incorporates at its origins the futural idea of parental love! It is thanks to 'fecundity' that relationships of love and care avoid closure and become as much 'impregnated with the future' as 'obsessed with the possibility of impregnation'. *Parental love for the third as child* - which predates the parents' own affair and prevents it becoming closed - thus implicates the 'I' with 'my other' (the lover) and with 'the other' (the child') in an anarchic way. 'My other' is 'the other whom I have already loved disinterestedly and obsessively - approaching him or her as unique and 'for me'. But in memory and re-presentation lies the danger that the emotional affair of the couple will be equated with inter-*esse* synchronism unless it is accepted that the engagement with 'the other' is larger than that with 'my other'. It is for this reason that sociality incorporates the idea of the third, the not-yet loved by the couple, in the form of a 'child'.

[3]Of course, we must bear in mind the particularity of Levinas' idea of responsibility *as* passivity. Bernhard Waldenfels explains that the 'traditional idea of responsibility means that wherever something is said and done, everybody speaks with his own voice and that in one's voice the universal voice of Reason also finds expression. The dialogical idea of responsibility (λογον διδοναι), inherited from the Greeks, meets with the juridical idea of imputation (*imputatio*) invented by the Romans. Thus somebody is responsible for something to somebody, *three instances taking part in the process of giving account.*' (Waldenfels in Peperzak ed. 1995: 40; my emphasis). Of these three instances the first is, for Weidenfels, that something is said or done *'for which* one is responsible. Here we are dealing with the results from saying or doing. The process of saying or doing coagulates into a state of affairs ... what Lévinas calls the said ... [where] everything is put in the perspective of the past' (ibid.). Secondly, we are responsible *'to somebody,* to a forum or a tribunal, which is more or less personal or anonymous ... words and deeds are regarded from the perspective of a neutral Third' (ibid.). From this trans-subjective standpoint of the Third what is said and done is transformed into an objective state of affairs subjected to objective standards 'with the effect that only reasons count and not opinions and wishes' (ibid.). Finally, 'somebody, being responsible has to justify *himself.* The state of affairs would be a mere fact and not deed if it could not be causally attributed to a certain or to several speakers. This attribution or imputation does not happen to the subject of speech and action

Lévinas' subjective 'desire' has little similarity to what is commonly denoted by this word.[4] The difference, in short, is 'disinterestedness', which characterises only 'ethical violence'. Lévinas believes that all desire is 'insatiable'. But non-intentional responsibility distinguishes between insatiable desire as obsession, and desire as 'want' or lack.[5] The violence of the desire for the other as unique is imposed by means of 'one-way acts of kindness', making up the 'gratuitous charity' which characterises the sociality of beings, who thus have more than a desire to be-with-each-other. The being-with-each-other, in other words, is sustained by the 'good' violence of acts of being-for-each-other, whereby the other is approached obsessively as more unique than different. It is thus through 'passion' and 'obsession' that the pre-intentional being 'opens-up' to its otherness *and* maintains alterity. But all this depends on responsibility being an individual passion.[6] What happens when responsibility is disconnected from compassion? It is then more difficult to accept that justice is the 'child' of charity and the product of love (OB: 43, 125, 126). Where Lévinas says that love 'must always supervise justice' (ibid.) he implies that there is, embedded in justice, an obsession with *disinterested charity* that must not be underestimated or thought to be 'separate from' and 'posterior to' the sober calculations of judgement. Such obsession is to be found inside the 'pathos of liberalism' for equality and fairness. Indeed the liberal pathos for equality and tolerance towards difference presupposes the obsession (and thus the 'good violence') with which the uniqueness of the other is claimed by each me. The implication for law is that 'subjectivity'- the individual subject of formal equality - must first be thought of as *free* to engage in unilateral actions of approach which open up a space otherwise than inter-*esse* for approaching each other-as-other.

Thus, it must be recognised that prior to discernment, comparison and calculation, the subject is, as it were, 'self-entitled' to the 'childish' obsession and erotic desire 'for an absolutely unique other'. The right to responsibility presupposes such a self-entitlement. Prior to assuming reciprocity with one another, subjects surprise each other through impositions and assumptions of responsibilities. Prior to the commitment to be fair with one another, beings must mark one another with the identity of absolute uniqueness. Prior to relating to my other person as inter-changeable with third others, I must enter proximity with

---

après coup. On the contrary, someone constitutes him- or herself as 'subject' by assuming responsibility ...' (ibid.).

[4] See my Introduction, n. 9.

[5] For Levinas (and, perhaps this constitutes his greatest difference from psychoanalysis) 'desire' for otherness precedes being's interest in the other's being and possessions. This is to say that the 'object' of my desire is *so* elusive that, at the end of the day, the movement from me to the other deserves to be described as absolutely 'one-way'. My desire for the other as unique is inessential and proceeds infinitely to claim his/her uniqueness without substantiating the claim. It is desire for the other as sign of Infinity.

[6] 'Radical youth' (HAH: 43), 'heteronomy' (DVI: 152), 'generous impulse' despite sobriety (NTR: 91): these are just some of the indicative expressions used.

him/her - that is, be exposed to him/her as incomparable and unique (ibid.). Prior to discerning the other's characteristics, or surrounding him/her with my projections, I am first myself bound to be obsessed with the other as if he/she were unique or 'the only one that matters'.[7] Detaching the other from all other reference but me is the self's non-selfish way of assuming responsibility. I come to assume my captivity by the other and act as their 'hostage'. In a sense I am an obsessive (and even psychotic?) stalker of 'the other', rather than merely an 'I' which commits itself to projections and abstractions towards others. It is important to stress that in Lévinas, the word 'freedom' is used interchangeably with 'being hostage'. Engaging in the 'good violence' of approach is therefore an inescapable obligation. It is for this reason that this 'violence' is redeemable; further, it is an opening to the eventuality of 'ineluctable surprise' for proximity, which entails the irreducibly astonishing experience of one's desire to be-for-the-unique-other, despite the fact that the other cannot ever be grasped by one's intentions. This relationship is constant surprise because it is not reducible to the inoffensive relationships in knowledge (where justice is thought to be separate from charity and love), nor to the 'adequational' relationships in exclusive love, without consideration for the third, without justice.

II
The law on the consent of the incompetent

> Is approach to be defined by commitment, and not rather commitment by approach? Perhaps because of current moral maxims in which the word neighbour occurs, we have ceased to be surprised by all that is involved in proximity and approach (OB:5).

> The responsibility for another is a saying *for* the other prior to anything said. The surprising saying ... is against the 'winds and tides' of being, is an interruption of essence, a disinterestedness imposed with good violence (OB:43).

Let me illustrate these points after making a thematic return to Common law. Law's understanding of the encounter between patients and doctors and other therapists is marked by emphasis on patient autonomy and consent.[8] The ways in which the judiciary construct the meaning and scope of patient consent is of great importance in the practice and theory of medical law. But an unproblematic emphasis on the autonomous patient obscures how, if at all, the liberal idea of

---

[7]Levinas' proximity as obsessive but disinterested approach resembles the detachment of the one who wears a cognitive 'veil of ignorance'. However, otherness in not an 'aspect' of my other which I happen to ignore; nor is it my other's 'dark', negative side or mortality; otherness stands for the unknowable *topos* from which the other questions me and captures my attention.

[8]It is only through obtaining a 'free and informed consent' that a doctor engaging in intrusive therapeutic actions escapes criminal and civil liability.

patient consent to medical treatment guarantees the fundamental human rights of patients with no consciousness or with severe mental disabilities. Here, I am focusing on patients whose consciousness is not extinguished but severely debilitated. The responsibility of doctors, relatives and often, judges to act unilaterally upon such patients is obscured if we remain in the realm of ideal doctor-patient reciprocity in the division of therapeutic labour. This is what happens at present in law, where the emphasis is put on so-called tests of patients' 'competency', that is, on tests which establish whether a patient is or is not capable of consenting to or refusing medical intervention. For most of this century lawyers did not need such tests, for patients' 'competency' was derived from their juridical 'status' (in turn, this was informed by medical/psychiatric assessments). Thus minors and mentally disturbed adults were automatically incompetent. However, we now accept that a patient's capacity to reject or consent to treatment must be presumed as 'of right', that is, irrespective of immaturity or mental impairment. Yet there are many instances in which those who assume the care of such patients wish to rebuff this presumption. In this respect several tests have been proposed for establishing whether a patient can exercise their right to refuse treatment. These include the 'reasonable outcome' test, whereby a court reviews the 'reasonableness' of the most likely outcome of the patient's choice. This test has been rejected by liberal lawyers as being potentially too 'subjectivist'. Further, there is the 'evidencing a choice' test whereby a patient must show that in refusing treatment he or she has made a proper 'choice', i.e. weighed the 'pros and cons'. This, too, has been rejected as too arbitrary. Why, after all, cannot a patient refuse treatment without having considered at all the implications of receiving no treatment?

Both these tests have by now supposedly been superseded by a third, whereby all patients need to show before being allowed to refuse treatment is that they 'understand' the nature and purpose of the medical treatment which is proposed to them. This more 'liberal' view is now officially embraced by the British state.[9] I argue, however, that this 'objective' test pays only lip service to the idea that patients' autonomy ought to 'transcend' their circumstances and not depend upon the 'rationality' of their choice, or even the existence of a genuine choice. The relevant legal literature recognises this to an extent, pointing to an ambiguity in law on whether the new test requires a patient to be generally capable of understanding, or merely to show 'actual understanding' in the event. In the former sense, the new test is nothing but a concealed version of the old status criterion. The preferred interpretation is that the patient ought to be expected to show no more than 'actual understanding' of their condition and the treatment proposed to them. Nevertheless, it can always be argued that even if the more liberal interpretation (i.e. 'actual understanding') was somehow entrenched, this would not prevent the judiciary from qualifying the 'reasonableness' of a patient's refusal (where the patient evidences a choice) nor oblige them to recognise the patient's right to

---

[9]Law Commission Consultation Papers 'Mentally Incapacitated and Decision-Making: A New Jurisdiction' (no. 128, 1993) paras 3.19-3.35.

refuse treatment with no proper choice. Therefore, there is justifiable concern that any legal test for 'competency' inevitably obscures the many considerations that weigh on judges' minds before they allow a patient to refuse treatment. Already in the 1970s, when the new approach began to emerge, the radical academic view was that the recourse to law by those who care for mentally vulnerable persons in order to provide an 'objective' test of competency compared with the search for the Holy Grail.[10]

I submit that the debate over the degree and timing of 'understanding' that the patient is expected to show before being deemed capable of exercising their autonomy is misleading. The real issue is how the responsibility of carers for their subjective reactions to the welfare of the mentally vulnerable is concealed behind malleable 'competence tests'. Moreover, I argue that if indeed there can be no respect for individual rights without the 'ethical violence' of prior one-way 'compassion', then the many 'competence tests' act to obscure this, with the result of introducing (potentially disastrous) falsely 'universal' truths about patients' rights. Case law verifies this view. For example, even where a minor suffering from anorexia shows that she 'actually understands' the nature of the proposed treatment (force-feeding), the court presumed that it is a feature of anorexia that the subject can no longer understand the importance of food.[11] In another example, an adult mentally handicapped woman was deemed incompetent to refuse and was sterilised 'in her best interests'. The test of 'actual understanding' of the purpose of treatment was not employed, albeit the woman was said to have the mental age of a six-year-old, i.e. an age where a girl can 'understand' the difference between 'having babies' and not having them.[12]

I propose, therefore, that the problem with the consent of the mentally vulnerable be dissociated from 'tests' which purport to establish whether a patient is competent. I agree that they must always be treated as if autonomous; for it is only through such a presupposition that the absolute of their person is recognised and their unique being is 'elevated' above the circumstances of their weakened, confused or non-existent consciousness. But it is important not to forget that this absolute uniqueness is not so much 'recognised' as *desired*. When a patient's consciousness is diminished or missing, his or her unicity does not 'depend', as it is often said, on 'certain basic biological functions' without which it would be 'permissible' to treat the comatose as already dead; nor does this unicity depend upon the ability of the patient to manifest signs of a weak but nevertheless still 'persevering' consciousness as the 'essence of human life'- the presence of which 'obliges us' to treat him or her as a fully autonomous person.

---

[10]'The search for a single test of competency is a search for a Holy Grail. Unless it is recognised that there is no magical definition of competency to make decisions about treatment, the search for an acceptable test will never end.' Roth, Meisel and Lidz, 'Tests of Competency to Consent to Treatment'; 134 *Am. J. Psychiatry* 279 [1977].

[11]*Re W (a minor)* [1992] 4 All E.R. 627.

[12]*Re F (a mental patient: sterilisation)* [1990] 2 AC 1.

How is it at all possible that a doctor or judge can respond to a duty to face the mental sufferer as unique despite the fact that the patient's consciousness recedes, so that the manifestation of individual difference gives way to anonymity? How can diminished consciousness not leave the patient a mere object for manipulation? The uniqueness of such an abstract being must be understood as the product of obsessive compassion of the subject of consciousness for the subject of diminished consciousness. Indeed, the human rights of the mentally vulnerable must exist independently of their actual circumstances and also from all entitlement - 'all tradition, all jurisprudence, all granting of privileges, awards or titles, all consecration by a will abusively claiming the name of reason' (OS: 117). Thus, to begin an encounter with the ill by recognising rights which are independent of conferral and deprivation entails a 'violent tearing loose' of the patient, first from the determining order of nature in which his or her existence is caught, and second, from the social structure in which his or her person is involved. The 'suspension of all reference' is a necessary price for expressing the alterity or absolute of every person. But it is a price worth paying, since the suspension of all reference does not extend to *me* - the me who holds myself *responsible*. It is a paradox that such violent responsibility should also secure the freedom of my absolute person - that which is incomparable, non-exchangeable and 'unique' beyond the individuality of multiple individuals, such as patients 'of the same kind'.

And how does the carer or judge redeem the violence of his or her 'obsessive' approach to the mentally ill? Compassion stands as a strange authority, older and higher than any other which at once binds and frees one to do so; it does not so much authorise anything, as obliges one to act as if this were authorised, thus implicating oneself in a responsibility for such violence. In short, it is authority-*qua*-responsibility for this violence which *justifies* the respect for the abstract rights of the other. Under this rubric, the determination to recognise autonomy even in the most horror-implicated patients can be thematised as the result of an obsessive, insatiable desire for compassion for the sufferer as other to the objectively/subjectively suffering patient. The 'object' of disinterested compassion is not the patient as 'different' from others yet ultimately a member of a class of similar individuals; but rather, an impatient and abstract sufferer who demands to be treated by someone who will see themselves as 'the one' with the 'right' to care for him/her as if he/she were the only one of his/her kind that mattered. In consequence, what carers 'ought to do' with respect to the medical treatment of such persons should not be inferred from the patient's objective and/or subjective interests. By contrast, the first question of justice which must be asked with regard to the treatment of such persons is, how to safeguard their 'right' to be treated by a *subjectively 'free'* subject who is called to be both bound to *and* responsible for his/her obsession and pure emotion. In other words, the case with the subject of diminished consciousness shows that:

> Responsibility for another is *not an accident* that happens to a subject but precedes essence in it, has not awaited freedom in which an engagement to another would have [already] been made. I have not done anything and I have always been under

accusation: persecuted. The ipseity ... is a hostage. The word *I* means *here I am*, answering for everything and everyone. Responsibility for the others that has not been a return to oneself, but an exasperated contracting, which the limits of identity cannot retain ... The responsibility for another, an unlimited responsibility which the strict accounting of the free and non-free does not measure, requires subjectivity as an irreplaceable hostage ... In the accusative, which is not the modification of any nominative - in which I approach the neighbor for whom, without having wished it, I have to answer, the irreplaceable one is brought out [*s'accuse*] (OB: 114).

I submit that in the case of incompetent patients, as in all cases, responsibility for the force by which this other is abstracted must not be hidden behind false authorities. In so far as the recognition of rights for the mentally vulnerable is linked to 'truth', either about their status or about their ability 'to understand', there is a deficit of judicial responsibility. Without personal responsibility for the unilateral act by which the mental patient is faced as other, so that he or she can be abstracted as an absolute rights-holder, the principles of patient autonomy and self-determination (which consent is meant to express) lose all sense and appear absurd and arbitrary. However, the judges' utterly individuated, non-shareable personal responsibility in their proximity to patients can reverse this situation. Through assuming responsibility as their only authorisation, a judge can uphold the incompetent patient's autonomy (or, more precisely, can impute autonomy to the patient) and shift the accusation of absurdity from the principles of law to the intrinsic absurdity of the patient's situation. After all, human suffering is, and must be responded to obsessively because it is totally absurd.

III
The shame

It is of the essence of judgment as fate that while the impact of judgment ... may escape codification and indeed may be inexpressible, it is nonetheless remembered and inscribed. *The soul of the judge is marked by judgment.* While others may not perceive or judge the act of judging, the judgment is indelible nonetheless: judgment (discrimination and taste) traces and defines the subject that judges, and the body carries the corpus or product of judgment. The eternal return is thus the return of the same in the substantive form of becoming or difference (Gilles Deleuze 1983: 25-29).

Let me examine closely the two American cases which pioneered the new legal 'competency test' in the 1970s (*Yetter* and *Northern*) and trace, in the words of Deleuze above, how the judgment 'marked the soul' of the judges.[13] The sixty-year-old Ms Yetter had spent the longest part of her life in an institution suffering from 'schizophrenia chronic undifferentiated'. When a routine physical

---

[13]Re Maida Yetter (1973) 96 D & C 2d 619 (CP Northampton County PA) and *State of Tennessee v. Northern* (1978) 563 SW 2d 197 (Tenn. CT App.).

examination indicated the possible presence of a carcinoma of the breast, the doctors recommended that a surgical biopsy be performed together with any additional, corrective surgery that would be indicated by the pathology of the biopsy. Ms Yetter opposed the treatment without explanations. When, however, her matter reached a court, the judges heard her objecting to the operation mainly because she was convinced that biopsy would have 'similarly' devastating effects on her to those her aunt had suffered in the past (although the aunt had had her ovaries removed, rather than a breast). 'Thereby' the biopsy on the breast would 'interfere with her genital system, affecting her ability to have babies'. Also, she was convinced that biopsy would necessarily lead to mastectomy, and that this would prohibit a 'movie career' which she was 'anticipating'.

The judges decided that in law Ms Yetter was not incompetent to refuse life-saving treatment. I have said earlier that the recognition of inalienable rights of the other human entails a paradoxical form of violence whereby we achieve their extraction from all reference so as to mark them with an absolute identity of uniqueness. Thus, it can be said that the court's decision in *Yetter* is an instance of judicial 'disinterestedness' towards Ms Yetter's existential circumstances which made possible their offer of compassionate relief to this patient as abstract 'sufferer' and subject of a-priori rights. However, the judges also went out of their way to stress that, during the hearing, Ms Yetter had appeared 'alert, interested and obviously meticulous about her personal appearance'. The problem is that, thus framed, the decision only seemingly enshrines the principle that the patient's right to refuse treatment exists independently of her mental illness and the outcome of her choice. For it appears that the court did not say that it allowed Ms Yetter to decide independently of her actual mental disability. According to the judges, her refusal of the biopsy before them had 'evidently' been made 'in a moment of psychological lucidity'- something which was not confirmed by forensic psychiatrists. In short, this case was framed in such a manner that the 'new' test of competency based on understanding only seemingly superseded the less desirable tests based on 'reasonableness' of choice and 'evidencing a choice'. In fact the new test can be seen as incorporating these other tests. Simply, in this case the patient's desires and the deadly consequences of her rejection did not stop the judges from granting autonomy on the basis that Ms Yetter had clearly made a choice. Further, the fact that in response to the specialist's evidence that death could follow if no treatment was given, the court felt obliged to reiterate that suicide is no longer illegal, suggests that the judges *did* in fact consider the consequences of the patient's choice. In this way the judges in *Yetter* broke their own law.

Yetter is far from a 'disinterested' approach to the rights of the mentally incompetent. The judges emphasised that the patient's meticulous appearance was 'consistent' with her desire to become a movie star.[14] Their compassionate

---

[14]For lawyers this is important both from the point of view of continuity of personality and of coherence in the various desires a subject articulates. There is an assumption that the identity of the patient survives their suffering intact if they show themselves to be the *same* person 'before and after' their illness.

recognition of that patient's right to refuse medical treatment, here, lacks disinterestedness towards her existential qualities. Relevant are Lévinas' categories of undifferentiated existence, anonymous existent and eponymous being, as they appear in his *De l'existence à l'existant* (DE 1947). When consciousness is suppressed under the burden of one's existence, in the sleep that follows a hard day's work but also in states which we call 'diminished consciousness', we cannot talk of 'one' as anyone in particular. The one who is embraced by sleep 'is there', although he or she does not actively exist. Of course as long as biology allows, the heart still beats, the lungs still inhale and there is still neurological activity, we may still talk of a particular 'existent', separated from anonymous, undifferentiated 'existence' by its own effort and perseverance. The compassion and concomitant responsibility of the carer does not increase or decrease in accordance with the other's existential activity. In fact responsibility presupposes that we approach the other as if unique irrespective of the activity of organic perseverance or the absence of it. Responsibility for the other's unique being must be independent of our fluctuating interest in the other's relative activity and passivity.   It is responsibility for a being suspended *there*, between sleep and waking, or a being exposed to the alternatives of activity and passivity. The other 'says': come to me in my sleep, or in my illness where only my body's effort still separates me from anonymous existence and, despite all my exposure, approach me gently, as if I were the only being that mattered. When one's consciousness is dormant or weak, if one's neighbour does not succumb to the desire to approach one as unique in the abstract, one's eponymous and singular being might be obscured by one's anonymous existence and treated accordingly. This is the essence of our complaint against those who 'kick us out of bed'. Alternatively, individuated being is equally obscured if one's conscious activity is falsely equated with one's existential struggle in persevering 'against all odds' or in enduring suffering.

Accordingly, in cases of insanity and depression it is important not to subject our respect for the sufferer's individuated being, and our concern for the concomitant demand they express, to their capacity or incapacity either to 'endure' or to render intelligible their suffering.   For then, the other's demand to be recognised as unique being is falsely equated to their existential ability to persevere or endure. Such false equation ultimately collapses a mentally disturbed being into its illness, and gives false license to irresponsible and abusive attitudes against it, such as pity and disgust. When the imputation of rights to mentally ill persons does not explicitly refer to the inescapable compassion that precedes and motivates it, it becomes a form of just such abuse. One is entitled to criticise the authors of such decisions, not for the ethical violence of their compassion, but for the different, deliberate, kind of violence of pity or disgust. The existence of such pity and/or disgust indicates that the disinterestedness towards the patient's own existential effort that both compassion and respect require has given way to the 'either-or' of interest/indifference towards that effort.

The way *Yetter* was framed fails to express its truth: that despite Ms Yetter's schizophrenia the judges *felt* obliged to recognise her as a unique subject of a right to refuse treatment independently of her psychological and physiological impairments. The judges did not so much evidence a moment in which the patient had 'clear understanding', as invite her to perform a show of understanding. The suffering that they witnessed was absurd. There was no better way to recognise this suffering and to extract Ms Yetter's person from all this absurdity, than to give her a moment in court in which she could 'act' that she understood. It was not that her performance in court showed understanding; rather, the performance was construed as 'understanding'. In this sense the true 'moment of lucidity' did not concern Ms Yetter but the judges. It was a moment in which all that mattered was their responsibility for the sufferer 'here and now', disconnected from her past and future. They were concerned for her suffering 'right now' and not for her future biological preservation or perishing, or for the survival of her identity as someone who had wanted in the past to become a 'movie star'. It was with such force that the right of Ms Yetter to refuse treatment would indeed be disconnected from all her circumstances.

The judges' false insistence that Ms Yetter had experienced a 'moment of lucidity' denies their compassion. It was as if Ms Yetter were capable of approaching the judges already as a unique being, and, from the supposed vantage point of 'momentary lucidity', enact herself as someone who 'has always desired to be a movie-star' (in the past) and who is free to commit suicide (in the future). The rule on incompetent persons' right to refuse medical treatment thus appears entirely 'theatrical'. The judicial emphasis on the patient's 'momentary lucidity' implies, falsely, that there is a distance between the patient as abstract subject of rights and the patient as sufferer subject to the horror of illness. Moreover, it implies that this is a distance that the patient must herself cover. Also, with all the emphasis the judges placed on the schizophrenic woman's 'meticulous appearance', it becomes nearly impossible to trace in their judgement the extent to which the horror and absurdity of human suffering had mattered in their decision.

The artificial disconnecting of Ms Yetter's refusal of treatment from her naturally inflicted suffering underestimates the effects of such suffering on her, and presents her as someone who could conveniently endure her affliction - if only 'momentarily' - and who could imagine compensations for her endurance - by not losing her breast she could still imagine becoming a 'movie star'. *Yetter* can be understood as a case of irresponsible compassion, that is, compassion which is denied its disinterestedness. Although 'disinterestedness' is something one can take personal responsibility for (how else can the subject of diminished consciousness be treated as if unique?), the selective interest in another's existential trouble must be justified by recourse to false 'truths'. Here, the false 'truth' was that Ms Yetter had risen above her condition through her own effort. In *Yetter* the judges turned away from the nakedness and exposure of a present, singular, sufferer who was also a subject of rights under the disguise of deluded schizophrenic. Instead, their starting point was her status as schizophrenic, to which they claimed a miraculous, momentary exception. Further, as the judges' emphasis on Ms Yetter's presence as 'alert, interested and obviously meticulous about her personal appearance' indicates, they conceived of a subject which supposedly could on its own invest its persona with, or divest its persona of, incompetence. It is for this reason that - contrary to the essence of their new test - Yetter's judges did look at the nature of her past desires and the future consequences of her decision.

Before the famous phrase 'Arise ... and walk' (Mark 2:9) Jesus had not condemned suffering as absurd but had related it to the sins that supposedly had brought it about. In *Yetter* too it was as if what was condemned was Ms Yetter's inability, before and after her 'moment of lucidity', to assimilate her suffering into an experience that she could reflect upon and understand. This situation is unacceptable. The framing of this decision denies that Ms Yetter was a sufferer - that is, someone who exists but has trouble being unique without help from others. Since the recognition of her right to refuse treatment was linked to her supposed ability to be herself - if only for a moment - it is as if the court were presuming her miraculous ability to come forth as a human being on her own: it is a case of 'Arise and walk'. However, although it can be argued that each human has a constitutional 'obligation' to exist (or, to keep with the Christian theme, to 'arise') there is no obligation to *be* ('... and walk' - but walk where? towards whom?). 'Being' is not like waking up to morning light in order to face life: it requires a different light, which is no less than the responsibility of other people. The individualisation of an existence which seems to be slipping into the obscurity of a clouded mind requires a certain violence on the part of its neighbour. Every human carries alone the burden of its existence, it perseveres and endures. But, the different burden of being unique weighs on the *neighbour's* shoulders. Justice to the sufferer requires individuated compassion, benevolence and empathy, all of which are described by Lévinas as individuated human 'vocations', disposing, in a political society, 'of a kind of extra-territoriality ... lucidity not limited to yielding before the formalism of universality (OS:123)' and not limited by natural determinism. Without these vocations in place, the protection of sufferers' absolute rights is amenable to deviations imposed in the name of 'necessity', with the same indifference to the other human that nature displays.

IV
The guilt

The inability of the judges to disconnect the issue of patient's rights to refuse treatment from the requirement that the patient must 'make a choice' is further highlighted by a comparison of this case with a similar subsequent one. A seventy-two-year-old Ms Northern had no specific mental disability other than old-age dementia. She was referred to a hospital by her neighbours with a case of severe gangrene. She refused life-saving surgery (amputation) but without offering any reasons. As she was sane one would have expected that her refusal of treatment would be recognised in law. This, after all, would have been the case even under the old, less liberal 'status' criterion. However, in court she was found to be incompetent to refuse the treatment. The court noted that 'she looks at [her feet] and insists that nothing is wrong with them' although they were 'evidently rotting and smelly'. Had she agreed that her feet were smelly and blackened, she would still have been allowed to reject medical treatment, and the court would not have judged the rationality of such refusal. Most importantly, however, the court also contrasted her case with the case of Ms Yetter and noted that Ms Northern, apart from her refusal to recognise that anything was wrong, had virtually nothing else to communicate to the court and gave no reasons for refusing medical treatment.

At this point it is worth mentioning that in Lévinas' phenomenology human 'suffering' is so abstract and incomprehensible that it does not offer itself for the description of what would be the 'object' of intentionality and will.[15] All illness pacifies the human beyond belief, overwhelming experience and consciousness. Suffering is a stranger to consciousness, inside consciousness. There can be no moment of 'understanding' suffering. The inability to perceive and represent suffering is not evidence of a 'failure' by perception and consciousness for which the sufferer is to be blamed. Thus Lévinas does not claim a martyr's sense, where suffering is an existential opportunity for self-transcendence. As far as the sufferer's self is concerned, suffering is useless. However, the sufferer's passivity turns into their neighbour's compassion. Lévinas rejects intellectualism according to which one's suffering cannot signify in another except through the limited categories employed by the mind. Instead, Lévinas insists that one's passively expressed suffering, as pure 'epiphany' and invocation of Face, ought to cause in the witness an obsessive compassion which traverses their consciousness 'counter-current-wise', and is inscribed in it as something foreign to it, as dis-equilibrium or delirium (OB: 101).

The silently ill, the comatose, and those who respond to their suffering with anger or self-abandonment cannot become mere objects in the eyes of the rest of us because, through the inevitability of violent compassion, we must still hypostasise them as unique recipients of our responsibility. They are subjects in a unique sense, perhaps absurdly even, as 'pure exposure', vulnerability and nakedness. The ethical subjectivity of the ill is secured by the fact that despite their sickness, their Face 'still speaks' with a voice which is supplication as well as demand. The uniqueness of the vulnerable other is not jeopardised by the absence of articulated desire and by the imminence of death, as long as we feel obliged to seize it as unique. Medical responsibility for every unique sufferer goes a lot further than merely doing what is possible to cure a body or appease an ego; judicial responsibility, too, extends further than merely respecting formal patient autonomy. Both these professions are underscored by vocational compassion, and desire to approach those who are at the brink of becoming anonymous as if unique. In the absence of God, this is also a desire to condemn the absurdity of naturally inflicted suffering. Yet, because of the absence of God, this desire to extract the sufferer from both nature and social order must be accompanied by a sense of infinite responsibility and bad conscience.

---

[15]For more see Chapter 3.

Ms Northern was deemed incompetent to refuse treatment for a more fundamental reason than that she 'looks at her feet and insists that nothing is wrong with them'. Unlike Ms Yetter, Ms Northern had not only rejected the 'objectivity' of the medical diagnosis, but had also declined the opportunity to pass a subjective judgement on her afflictions, and failed to give any reasons why non-treatment would be better than treatment. Ms Northern had expressed her suffering silently, passively, without subsuming it under any considerations and calculations of treatment benefits versus benefits of no treatment. She showed that she could not take responsibility for the horrific, absurd and utterly unjustifiable suffering that nature had inflicted on her. It was entirely left to the judges to assume this responsibility and act. *Northern* bears the repercussions of the irresponsibility which surrounded the birth of the new, more liberal 'competency test' in *Yetter*. That test, based upon patient 'understanding', allowed the judges in *Yetter* to invite that patient to act at least as if she had 'understood': such are the obsessive results of the liberal pathos with uniqueness. But the pathos was concealed, as the invitation to the patient to 'act' that she understood became presented as an inference of an ability to understand. It appears, therefore, that there is still a critical 'choice' that the patient is expected to evidence, before being allowed to refuse treatment. What is critical is no longer the reasonableness of the choice between treatment and the alternative, illness and health, life and death. Under the new liberal test for competency these aspects are now a matter of complete indifference. But this is not yet meeting the standard that the patients' rights exist independently of everything. In fact the court in *Northern* appears to have made the right to refuse treatment subject to an existential requirement: the patient must take a pro-active attitude towards his or her suffering. They must speak 'of it' - whether reasonably or not. But this is no less than obliging the sufferer to cover their horrific nakedness, vulnerability or destitution.

In the *Book of Job* the suffering of illness is repeatedly depicted in all its absurdity, arbitrariness and unjustifiability. But in the beginning Job's comforters insist on engaging him in a dialogue directed towards giving his sufferings a 'theodicy' meaning. They excuse themselves: 'if we assay to commune with thee, wilt thou be grieved? but who can withhold himself from speaking?' (at 4:2), and then persecute him so that he may remember possible reasons why he suffers, and anticipate future compensations. They do not care for the present Job who says: 'I cry out of wrong, but I am not heard: I cry out aloud, but *there is* no judgment' (19:7). Job's comforting neighbours demand from him a 'constructive' attitude; they want him to pretend that there is judgment to be made about his suffering. In other words, the comforters refuse to supply Job's suffering with the meaning of their responsibility. Job is self-exposed as a being about to give up - which, in the biblical context, amounted to losing face before God by 'cursing the day he was born'. This is something the 'comforters' would not face.

Today's equivalent of losing face before God is given by Lévinas in his idea of 'existence without existent': the human, on its own, perseveres in its existence, thus becoming by his/her own effort a separate existent. But the uniqueness of a human being does not result directly from this effort, nor from the recognition of this effort by others. The uniqueness of being is expressed in the hesitation between slipping into anonymous existence and becoming a separable existent; between remaining in the embrace of sleep in the morning and waking up to smell the coffee. Our disinterestedness towards these two poles frees us to face the unique being that lies between the two poles in its hesitation, in its tiredness, where the exhaustion with 'having to live' is not yet incorporated by the will to be left alone or cease to exist. There is a price to be paid for our freedom to face the suffering other as unique irrespective of the degree to which he or she slips into diminished consciousness, and, conversely, independently of the degree to which his or her consciousness still perseveres. This is our responsibility for our compassion: responsibility with no excuse and for no fault, including responsibility for one's compassion, which might also be called a persecution. This responsibility for the other's vulnerability and nakedness must not be understood in reverse, as if it were dependent on the degree to which the other either still 'hangs in there' or, alternatively, 'has already given up'. For then our compassion becomes abusive pity or disgust; then, the suffering other is asked to cancel their hesitation, their tiredness, on penalty of being called lazy and abandoned. This is what happened in the *Northern* case, where the judges, disgusted with the patient's rotting feet and with pity for her passivity, ordered the amputation.

Job's visitors come to him intrusively. They take him by surprise, compelled by their own compassion - under no authority but their own responsibility. Bad consciousness and irrevocable responsibility is the price to be paid for calling out Job's unique person just as he seemed to be losing it. It is a paradoxical form of violence which extends to the modern determination to recognise a right to refuse treatment to patients independently of their absurd circumstances. But when, as in the case of Job's comforters, the guiltless responsibility for the ineluctable violence of compassion is denied, then guilt for the deliberate violence of another sort is substituted. Job's comforters abused him by repudiating his anger, just as the judges of Ms Northern abused her by repudiating her silence. Job complained, 'I am as one mocked of his neighbour' (12:4). And, as if anticipating Ms Northern, Job's anger gives way to silence:

> Oh that my grief were thoroughly weighed, and my calamity laid in the balances together! For now it would be heavier than the sand of the sea: therefore my words are swallowed up (6:2-6:3).

V
'Empathy'

In this regard, let me insist upon the passive nature of the idea of granting rights as *compassion*. It is noteworthy that Lévinas does not subscribe to Husserl's transcendental theory of so-called 'empathy'. Husserl assumed that in empathy I do less than intend the other: I 'apperceive' the other as 'necessarily *alter*' to my *ego*. Nevertheless, from the point of view of ethics of alterity, this 'apperception' still places the other in a commonly shared space; it is as if the other 'ha[s] spatial modes *like* those I should have ... if I should go over there and be where he is' (Husserl 1950: 53). This formulation entails an extension of objective space and time, which, supposedly, I and my other share. As such, Husserl's 'empathic' solidarity contrasts sharply with Lévinas' thesis that the being-for-each-other requires a radical subjective de-positioning or dis-situating. For, in empathy:

> The unity of analogy replicates a unity or community which drags us in, gathering us together as though we were galley slaves chained one to the other, constituting a proximity devoid of meaning. Any effort to undo this conjunction and conjuncture would be heard only as a creaking of chains (OB: 279).

All in all, the world is encountered as irrepressibly and incessantly spontaneous and intimate even from within humanism and liberalism. But this is so, not through the existence of God nor due to the possibility of people engaging in inoffensive 'empathy', overcoming their egoism, but through the 'ethical violence' with which the self must approach its other as unique. This situation is beyond the subject's intentionality and/or empathic 'apperception', possibly it is also beyond religious faith. It is 'obsession'. The subject of obsessive desire for uniqueness is indifferent to all *situ*ation and geometry that 'precede' and 'situate' its other. It is paradoxical that in proximity I become attached through *detachment* rather than empathy. But otherwise, if we stay within the parameters that Husserl set for empathy, the beauty of the world as incessant event is lost. In his phenomenology, subjectivity is ultimately equated with consciousness and so it becomes an 'eon', i.e:

> self-possession, sovereignty, *arche*. All unpredictable aspects of its experience are revealed in advance ... accommodated to the shape of existing knowledge, and thereby rendered incapable of provoking absolute surprise (TI: 14).

It is only thanks to its 'obsession' that the subject relates to its other as an *unquenchable* source of responsibility which can never be discharged or de-limited. In the midst of the city, people still face each other as unique. In my every turning towards the face of the passing stranger (later I shall be invoking the relevant Greek term *pros-opsis*) I am caught in proximity with the other as that whom I desire to be 'the one for me' in both the ethical sense (i.e. the one for *my responsibility*) and the erotic one. This other that I desire is not just an imaginary 'construction' by myself, because confronted with the stranger, who is only fleetingly apparent and present, my self-consciousness is *shattered*. Who can 'I' be before the utter stranger whose anonymity and undifferentiated position in the crowd (let alone the mortality which makes him or her stranger to the world!) engages my consciousness but leaves it disinterested? With regard to the stranger of whom I know nothing, but nevertheless desire, consciousness is *restlessness* ('are they *for me*?' I wonder) and *interrogation* ('who must I become for them?'). The disinterested if brief encounter with the stranger in the crowd does not cause my 'alienation' (before the non-interesting I have no self to be alienated from), but my dis-situation.

The 'good violence' connected with human contact of which I talked above is needed to express this ordinary adventure of inter-subjectivity before each of the many surprising others of a day. In order to express this adventure, I claim 'my other' to be unique. In Lévinas the irreducible 'surprise' of face-to-face proximity is *not* lacking in large human associations and impersonal gatherings (the former constitutes the 'diachrony' of the latter). The compassion and love of personal responsibility (the singular desire to be-for-each-other-as-the-one-for-my-responsibility) may *appear strange* ideas to those who equate 'justice' with the legal order of intersubjectivity which obscures the anarchy of the face-to-face. Charitable responsibility 'for nothing' may well continue to be thought of as separate from justice, in so far as the latter is reduced to those principles which allow for the preservation, measurement and calculation of our meaningful and conflicting desires to be 'with' each other. This situation relates to matters which I examined in Chapter 1. The self encounters its obligations in the other's Face, in an experience of incommunicable 'revelation' and epiphany.[16] How to describe the surprising event of facing another as *my* other? I would need to avoid presenting the event of revelation as a mere 'manifestation' in which I am bound to present both myself and my other *anachronistically* as if we were co-present. In the last case the presence of otherness in the same would then be reduced to the simulation of an 'origin' by the same. Such is the difference between Lévinas' alterity and Derrida's complementary notion of 'strange phenomenological symmetry' between me and my other (see Derrida 1967, but also his 'The Mystical Foundation of Authority' in M. Rosenfeld *et al.*, eds. 1992). Derrida commits just such an error by abstracting a relationship of adequacy and correspondence from the *irreducible* tension which exists in reality between the counter-experience of alterity and its simulation by re-presentation for the purpose of accounting to third others and rendering visible my dealings with the other. To be sure, the triangular relation of 'specularity' (me and other as seen by the third) surrounds proximity; proximity cannot be lived 'secretly' and 'spontaneously'; it becomes mediated, and something that the subject must symbolise or simulate. But, this is still only *my* responsibility and problem, not my other's. This point is important in relation to Derrida's view that in the asymmetry of the face-to-face there is also a strange symmetry due to the fact that 'I know my self to be the other of another' (Derrida 1967: 188).

---

[16]Again, it cannot be overstressed, this experience is unlike the appropriational relationship of knowledge (as a measure of abstract adequacy or correspondence) nor is it a mere relation of desire (as a mimetic identification as a dual impulse of being in and having the same time and space). The other concerns me - and is 'desired' by me in Levinas' sense - *because* I must claim him/her to be unique and, thus, pay less attention to who he/she appears to be or what he/she appears to have.

Proximity resembles a see-saw on which I am affected by and respond to the weight of my other even if am unaware and ignorant of our mutual placement and weight; I am not yet 'playing' because I am responding passively, involuntarily and without any interest whatsoever. I am responding solely by claiming that 'on the other end there is my unique other' with the force (or in Lévinas' terms, with a redeemable 'violence') which is commensurate to my other's otherness. No pleasure or satisfaction comes out of this, although there is the pure *enjoyment* of surprise! But if I come to think of this *as play*, from a third standpoint, I am already preparing to see the see-saw as a pair of scales with its own determinism and laws. What, then, is there to share with my 'third others' from this relationship of disinterestedness and play-less enjoyment with my other? In what way does the ethics of face-to-face proximity concern large human associations and its politics and laws? When I describe how a new friend is 'unlike anyone else I've met', I am unable to bring any convincing evidence. The suspicion looms in my audience that I am probably committing some abstraction of the other which will soon be upturned. But the well-meaning listening others will let me go on anyway. Why? Because in my delirium, or unsubstantiated Saying about my other's uniqueness, they find hints of a desire for a society whose pluralism is guaranteed, but which is 'a non-additive multiplicity of unique beings' (HS 1987: 177). In such an utopian society the manufacturing of comparable difference with limited rights would not constitute the aim, but merely the means for expressing - by default! - the surprising impact of proximity.

Thus, I come back to the second type of rights-related 'violence' which Lévinas distinguishes. In so far as I do not recognise the obsessive violence of my claim that my other is unique and I see myself and my other from a neutral standpoint, as if we were always on scales rather than a see-saw, the ethical significance of proclaiming my others' uniqueness is lost. It ceases to perform the ethical act of referring to a 'lost utopia' (not a 'lost paradise') and calling for its re-assertion. This in itself constitutes an unnecessary and unjustifiable act of violence. Without surprise, human proximity and mutual 'servitude' appear either as slavery or simply as a voluntarily undertaken commitment. 'Free' subjects are thought to be the ones who take refuge in the symmetry and order of the law in order to escape this 'slavery' of proximity. But in so far as rights serve me only to express proximity-*qua*-commitment to the other or freedom from the other, the question of interest arises. The third asks me, why do I desire my 'new friend' to be unique? To answer this question is to betray my other. No matter what answer I may give it will seem that I desire the other as unique because he or she *has* more or less of whatever is valued according to a singular law or economy of desire. Moreover, to answer requires a work of collection, presentation and interpretation of phenomena. In doing so, I partake in the time in which the truth of beings' Being manifests itself, and which is called by Lévinas 'ontological'. This is the time of the boredom of practical and intellectual life which is taken over by the synchronic deployment of selfish interests or needs. These are the *same* between multifarious and different, but ultimately 'additive' (as opposed to unique) beings which exist 'without surprise', and Being is thought of as:

invincible persistence in essence, filling up every interval of nothingness which would interrupt its exercise. *Esse* is inte*r-esse*; essence is interest (OB: 4).

We must seek to find the difference between time lived as synchronic deployment of essence, on the one hand, and time felt as diachronic surprise - disinterested, involuntary implication by the neighbour, on the other. The latter constitutes the patience and passivity of the former. The deployment of essence and interest is as active as it is 'arrested'. Time keeps still and a moment is eternal, even if lived as mundane. 'Mundane' is the epithet that people with little patience throw back at time 'in revenge', as they realise the absurd infinity of their responsibilities and the infinite patience required. It characterises particularly large 'collectivities' or gatherings. Inside commerce, peace is boredom. Each being collects itself and its other in a unity through memory (retention and protention). This is a tautologous movement of simultaneous dispersion and recollection into presence of self and other. The beings which are mutually implicated through interest and pursue the satisfaction of their needs collaboratively but, essentially, each-for-itself, are additive units of an all-encompassing Same social totality (society). It is a time of monotony and boredom ('we're all the same ...') when all things are synchronised by theoretical views and projects. Therefore, when being is identified with its 'vital' active essence and interest to be-for-itself but 'with' others, in fact no particular being is identified but, instead, a distinct system is pronounced in which all beings are ordered.

CHAPTER 3

Medicine, Law
and the Non-sense of Suffering

Suffering is the evil of passivity, a passivity which is greater than all our corresponding power to act or endure. Strictly speaking one cannot even be conscious of one's own suffering. In circumstances of pure adversity consciousness is not an 'activity': it is rather an *undergoing* of passivity that is an undergoing of an undergoing. For there is no content in the 'being conscious of suffering' - just passivity which comes *despite consciousness*. This passivity - as a modality of being - signifies a quidity of being, and perhaps, a place whence comes the original signification of passivity, independently of its conceptual opposition to any activity. In this modality, being is abstracted from its psycho-physical conditions; in pure phenomenological terms, therefore, the passivity of the being which undergoes suffering is not the 'reverse' of some activity - as is the sensory receptivity which correlates to ...'object' which affects and impresses it. The passivity of suffering is more profound than that of the receptivity of the senses - the latter being already the activity of...perception. In suffering, sensibility is more passive than perceptiveness; it is pacification and ordeal that tries experience. It is evil *par excellence*; sensibility in suffering is being put on trial. It is not so much that passivity describes 'evil', it is rather that the undergoing of evil is understood as the passivity of being (EN: 108; my translation; my emphasis).

[The fact that suffering is 'absurd' poses] the primordial and inevitable problem with succour as *my duty*. Is not the horror [*le mal*] of suffering - extreme passivity, impotence, abandonment and solitude - also the non-assumable and therefore, through its non-integration in the unity of order and of sense, the possibility of there being a surety, a cover [*une couverture*] over a complaint, a loud cry, a groan or sigh, [as] original call addressed to me to provide relief, assistance, to come to the other's aid [?] [M]e whose alterity and exteriority promise [my other] health? [With this we come to the event of] Original Opening [as exposure to] ... pure suffering through a demand for analgesia [which] through the groan, [is] more overbearing, more urgent than a demand to console or to stave off death ... [In relation to] pure suffering, [as] intrinsically non-sensical and condemned, a *beyond* is formed *inside* the inter-human (EN: 109-10; my translation; my emphasis).

I
Suffering as non-phenomenon

Lévinas insists that in its immediacy suffering is an absurd irruption in being, a 'counter-occurrence' of experience and intentionality.[1] Thus 'suffering' designates being as radically passive, and as otherwise than a being of experience and intentionality. Paradoxically, this radically passive state expresses the unicity of the sufferer's 'self' more than activity or absence of activity of being without suffering, i.e. being which is attempting and experience all. If, as Lévinas says, suffering is ultimately 'absurd', then to witness someone suffering is to risk an encounter with pure non-sense. That 'I' must become responsible for the other's absurd suffering also entails becoming responsible 'for nothing', neither with interest nor with indifference. Therefore, 'I' can engage with the adversity my other is undergoing *only* through 'disengagement'. This conception of inter-subjectivity points to the opposite of *esse,* that is, essence and persistence in Being where one's self is 'different' from another's but not unique. The 'nakedness' of the subject of absurd suffering points to its ineluctable, passive exposure to the otherwise than being/non-being. Of what 'consists' the radical passivity of the sufferer and the one who witnesses it? Let us think of delirium and an excessive cry for help. A cry affects us with equal authority whether it calls us to a hypochondriac, a 'childish' adult or a cancer patient. Each sufferer - including those suffering with self-inflicted wounds - must be approached as 'the only one that matters' without reason; equally, let us think of the pure emotion of the survivor before the dead, their crying 'for nothing' which exceeds the 'function of mourning'. Unlike eulogies, the survivor's tears do not attempt to fill the void opened by the other's disappearance but merely mark the place where the other stood before, reserving his or her a 'place under the sun', even when he or she is absent. And so, at least following Lévinas' thought, 'human suffering' neither alienates nor brings people closer: absurd suffering calls for disinterested obsession and engagement through disengagement.

A few clarifications are needed here concerning Lévinas's own phenomenology of 'suffering', which he begins with a look at the classic school of

---

[1]It must be stressed that when Lévinas refers to the passivity of 'inassumable', 'useless' or absurd suffering he is not alluding to an 'excess' of an intense sensation that one can longer bear nor to a quantitative excess that opposes and overcomes the measure of our sensibility and the perceptive means available to our consciousness. Indeed it is because we tend to think of extreme suffering in terms of *excess* that we are often inclined to see certain incurable conditions as 'exceptional'. Rather, adjectives such as 'inassumable', 'absurd' etc. serve to remind that *all* suffering comes *despite* experience and despite consciousness. The horror of illness is not measurable according to the degree to which it tries the patient's greater or lesser powers of 'endurance'. Rather its horror lies in suffering which *always* comes despite the limits of patience. Suffering is thus always more than the subject can take.

phenomenological analysis of illness, initiated by Husserl, which had focused only on the plurality of meanings of 'suffering'.[2] These meanings were sought within the self-consciousness of either the sufferer or the external witness. However, in his chapter on *useless* suffering (*La Souffrance Inutile*) Lévinas distinguishes the ethical significance of illness-suffering, which he maintains to be absurd non-sense, from the 'meaning' it receives as sensory/psychological 'content' in the patient, e.g. as pain and discomfort, and its cognitive meaning (EN: 107-19) e.g. as symptom of pathology. The so-called 'experience of suffering' of either the subjective sufferer or the objective witness in fact conceals an indefinite group of disparate emotional experiences which cannot be grouped together in a unified experience nor be known. Instead, we refer to the suffering body as undergoing a 'pre-original' experience of suffering in which it finds itself trapped. Prior to referring to the sufferer as a sensory receiver - a body that experiences suffering - and/or as an intentional sense-bestower, we must first understand it in its *extreme passivity* where the subject is indistinguishable from object. In this sense the sufferer too is a *disengaged witness* to his/her own unintelligible suffering, but of course, not an indifferent witness.

Similarly, the external witness of suffering is not only 'experiencing' the sufferer's expressions of pain and discomfort. More importantly he or she remains unable to bestow a meaning on this event of horror. The absurd expression of suffering can be witnessed irrespective of the patient's activity and/or inertia, endurance or stoic acceptance. The witness encounters the sufferer first of all as all-passive, expressing a demand for succour, otherwise than as a sovereign subject. However, this radically passive other cannot be reduced to a therapeutic 'object' by the intentional focus of the witness. Thus, the engagement with another's suffering (and the assumption of responsibility for it) is *independent* from the commitment one may or may not make towards it, for one is concerned for suffering one can neither comprehend *nor* ignore. Concern is not dependent on my relative interest in the eidetic kind of of suffering I am 'witnessing', always with horror. All in all, Lévinas depicts subjectivity's relation to the otherness of suffering (be it the external suffering of another *or* my own) in terms of *counter-intentionality*. Although eventually, consciousness either comes to assume the suffering it witnesses as a mere 'internal'/'external' object, or gives up and dies or 'despairs', the subject of consciousness must also be seen as ethically capable of transcending the passivity of suffering or of witnessing suffering.

Whilst suffering occurs 'despite' consciousness, the subject of consciousness strives to exist as it were 'in spite' of it. It wishes to contract, to coincide with itself as 'interiority' in remaining intact, ordered and active in the face of

---

[2]Except Husserl 1970 and 1964, and Merleau-Ponty 1962; for a particularly thorough phenomenological analysis of various aspects of the illness-experience, see Toombs 1988, 1990, 1992; Scarry 1985; Schutz and Luckmann 1973; Zaner 1964 and 1993; Kleinman 1988; Cassell 1979, 1982; Schwartz and Wiggins 1988: 137-71.

suffering which it assumes to be the effect of 'external' intrusions; in short consciousness pretends a heroic ability to assimilate the impact of suffering into its experience and knowledge. Thus, acting 'in spite' of suffering, consciousness aspires to an order of existence 'without exception, without disorder' (EN: 133). Going beyond this self-deception, Lévinas' account stresses the ineluctable sense-lessness, unintelligibility and absurdity of subjectivity's encounter with suffering - indeed this is one of the reasons why his essay is called 'Useless Suffering' - and points to how this useless suffering eludes the economy of closure and contraction by the subject of the dual instincts (or drives) to reproduce or die. Lévinas derives important lessons from subjectivity's exposure to such expressed but non-assumable absurdity. It is in useless, absurd suffering that each being remains *unique*. And it is in response to absurd, and utterly unjustifiable suffering that the external witness can care for the suffering other *as* other. Responsibility and guilt even for suffering one has not caused and cannot comprehend or even empathise with: these are the conditions in which ethical subjectivity learned to approach another being as unique. As such, the witness of suffering is the subject of an anarchic (not even empathic) compassion which does not wish to cancel the alterity with the other. This subject is neither active nor passive. The witness of suffering (who survives the absurdity of being affected by the other's suffering without comprehending it or doubting it) is moved 'counter-clockwise', or 'despite himself'. That is, it is in the exposure to my other's absurd suffering that I come to contract my ethical responsibility *for nothing*. In this connection, neither classic phenomenology nor existentialism had the analytical means or the interest to ascertain this engagement through disinterestedness of the human subjectivity with suffering.[3]

---

[3]Existentialism described the process of phenomenological reduction of one's absurd suffering through experience and knowledge as an inescapable self-alienation. J.-P. Sartre thus observed that, if I reflect on my pain and attempt to apprehend it, the pain ceases to be 'lived-pain' and becomes 'object-pain' (Sartre 1956: 440-441). Further, at the level of reflection illness represents an 'objective disease' which is known by means of bits of knowledge acquired from others (ibid. 466). This, I argue, is conceptually wrong, because at the level of first-hand undergoing of suffering there is not yet a unified 'self' to be alienated *from*. Rather, the disparity between undergoing and experiencing suffering indicates a *disjunction* between two very distinct analytical kinds of subjectivity each producing its own type of phenomenon. From an ethics point of view, the patient is not a self but an *object of* inassumable suffering, pure subjection, vulnerability, patience or else exposure. And yet, in the ethical sense I gave above, this strange living object which exists in pure exposure with no self-coincidence *also* remains a significant *subject* in relation to others. Thus even a comatose patient still concerns others as a significant subject. Others cannot relate to him/her as a phenomenological object (for example of pain). And so face-to-face with an absolute other they come to realise the first form of proximity. The ambiguity and scepticism that 'plague' the care of the comatose is no less than an instance of ethically inescapable 'substitution' for the other whose living status is indeterminate.

It is my argument that in the realm of so-called 'medical law', more than any other area of law, at stake is not merely liability for intentional or reckless causation of 'harm' but responsibility towards suffering one has not 'caused'. It should, therefore, be apparent at least in this area of law that responsibility for sufferings occurs gratuitously ('for nothing'). I argue in this connection that doctor-patient 'conflicts' (including those which are virtually legally constructed, as in cases where the incompetent patient's interests are represented by the Official Solicitor) could become the 'back door' through which the ethical (infinite) sense of *anarchic* responsibility of the being-for-each-other could re-enter the austere and repetitious realm of adjudication. If, in general, adjudication presumes a set of rules and principles of lawful conduct and then concentrates on interpretations of the meaning of the disputed 'object', e.g. the 'aim of treatment', medical adjudication finds itself exposed to the peculiar situation where such rule and principles must be asserted, arguably, despite an apparent *absence of meaning* of suffering. However, I submit that medical law at present seems unable to perform this role. Judges seem intent on bestowing on medical 'responsibility' the ordinary meaning this word has in law, *in spite of* the absence of meaning, or, in the terms of my Chapter 2, by 'appropriating' the absurdity of human suffering. In consequence, I argue, medical legal doctrine constitutes a blatant denial of the fact that responsibility is rooted in a diachronic 'non-intentional affectivity' of the sort that obtains in the witnessing of and obsessive compassion towards my other's suffering. In the process, a delimited idea of 'suffering' is instituted, making possible deviations from patients' human rights ascribed to necessity linked with pragmatism.

II
In the matter of the right to procreate

Let me illustrate the above. Alongside abortion-related issues, applications seeking legal sanction for non-consented sterilisation of mentally incompetent women provide the most important test of judicial willingness or reluctance to uphold the fundamental human right to reproduce in general, and women's reproductive rights in particular. Further, when such applications concern adult women the judicial responsibility in such matters is only accentuated. For judges cannot simply rely on medical opinion but must make up their own minds as to the mentally handicapped woman's actual capacity to consent to medical operations, and for that matter sterilisation. It is important whether in deciding this matter judges end up 'denying' or 'forfeiting' this fundamental human right

---

The emotional pain felt by those who cannot alleviate the extreme pain in certain illnesses is similarly no less than the realisation of pure proximity whereby the carer must first suffer *in the place* of the other.

(perhaps and/or 'sexed' right). Procreation - whereby one becomes responsible for another being - is an important way in which a being shows its *humanity-qua-right-to-responsibility*. The question of an incompetent woman's 'inalienable right to reproduce' is thus inextricably linked to another much more important one: does the woman's humanity transcend her mental incompetence as far as the rest of us are concerned? Is *humanity-qua*-responsibility-for-another-being dependent on the willingness and mental capacity of the potential parent? Whether we admit that the 'right to become responsible for a new being' exist *despite* the parent's consciousness, is crucial for whether we can conceptualise our own *obsessive* responsibility to help the incompetent exercise her right to become parentally responsible for another being.[4]

In England, the existence of the right to reproduce weighed heavily in the significant case of *Re D (a minor) (wardship: sterilisation)*.[5] A minor of eleven years of age suffering from Soto's syndrome and with an IQ of about 80 was found on evidence to have a '... fair academic standard with some prospects of improvement in her condition whilst her ability to marry and raise a child could not be discounted'. Judge Heilbron refused to allow the sterilisation. Her judgement includes the view that the operation involved the deprivation of a 'basic human right', and therefore:

> ... it would, if performed on a woman for non-therapeutic reasons and without her consent, be a violation of such right' (at 332).

---

[4]In Lévinas parental love is thus elevated to a higher principle governing the relationship between being-for-each-other (without a thought for the third, without discrimination, comparison and so without judgement) and being-with-each-other i.e. inter-*esse* and synchrony between beings as entities which persist individually in the totality of Being. The crucial reason is that in the one-way act of parental love we understand better how the self can be totally transcended by a unique other (whom it is obsessed with) *and* retain its identity as individual member of a totality of many 'others'. In the relation to the idea of 'child' the parental ego is not destroyed although it does become 'a stranger to itself'. The subject/object divide is thus radically subverted in the idea that one can relate to the other person as both different and part of one's self, by imitating parenthood. In conceiving the idea of 'child', the 'adult' (irrespective of their will and/or ability to conceive biologically) is not merely attempting to duplicate his or her self, but opens up to the idea of infinity. 'Fecundity' is the relation of the self called 'adult' with itself as stranger. In the actual feeling of parental love (which, however, is to be found in every human who cares for another) the adult comes, thus, to transcend the realm of the possible and to respond to a future 'not yet' which nevertheless matters to him- or herself now. The future which the child represents and the parents comes to conceive thereby, escapes the logic of continuity from past and present. (See Lévinas' chapter on 'Fecundity' in Tal.)

[5]*Re D (a minor) (wardship: sterilisation)* [1976] 1 All E.R. 326.

Naturally that judgement has since won acclaim.[6] In its aftermath it would have been settled, one imagines, that the misfortune of mental incompetence should not provide a basis for denying a person or a class of persons access to rights held to be inalienable. Yet it has since become standard practice for English courts on the one hand to praise *Re D* whilst on the other denying its most significant, if implicit, achievement: the recognition of a right to reproduction/responsibility independent of circumstances. *Re D* bore the seeds of its double reception. Judge Heilbron had stopped short of fully recognising such a right for mentally incompetent women. What featured prominently in the judge's opinion was the irreversibility of the operation on a girl whose 'prospects of mental improvement could not be discounted'. In short, what admittedly counted towards her decision was not the actual right to reproduce *as* incompetent, but the possibility that, in time, the girl's intelligence might have increased and she might have come to understand the implications of irreversible sterilisation with 'devastating effects'. It was in relation to such 'reasoning' that, ten years later, the House of Lords decided *Re B (a minor) (wardship: sterilisation)* by allowing the enforced sterilisation of another incompetent minor, B.[7] Nowhere in *Re B* was the principle challenged that 'nothing else but the ward's interests' should be considered in such decisions. There was no mention of the interests of the public and third-party interest in preventing childbirth where the mother is unlikely to care for the child, or where pregnancy and birth would place additional burdens on those who already cared for the mentally handicapped mother - that is, the court is supposedly not 'interested' in the parties that *initiated* the ward proceedings in order to secure a ruling that she may be sterilised; nor in the emotional distress that B's labour might cause to her carers and family. It was accepted on psychiatric evidence that B, a seventeen-year-old with a severe mental handicap, and an epilepsy sufferer, 'would never be able to give informed consent to medical treatment of any kind'. 'Therefore', the 'irreversibility' of the proposed sterilisation would not jeopardise any future consent and should not stop the operation from going ahead.

Justified thus, *Re B* is not expressing the limiting effects of B's illness which prevent her from fully assuming her 'involuntary' and 'disinterested' desire to be responsible for another human being. In consequence the decision cannot match the situation with the appropriate ethical sense of responsibility in those implicated in B's care. Rather, the judgment seems to rely on B's mental passivity

---

[6]The judgement of the Canadian Supreme Court in *Re Eve* [1986] 31 DLR (4th) 1, a case often referred to in and compared with English law, quoted *Re D* with approval and acknowledged the 'great privilege of giving birth' and the 'grave intrusion on a person's rights...which ensues from non-therapeutic sterilisation without consent' (at 32 per La Forest).

[7]*Re B (a minor) (wardship: sterilisation)* [1987] 2 all E.R. 206 Re Eve (1986) 31 DRL (4th) 1.

in order to deny such responsibility. B's suffering and passivity seem to have been of legal interest only in a particularly negative sense. Characteristically, Judge Bush found on evidence that sterilisation is needed in the 'best interests' of B given that the 'only' alternative to sterilisation would be to restrict further her freedom of movement. In this connection when Dr Barrow, a consultant expert contracted by the Official Solicitor, pointed the court to the obvious alternative of contraception, the judge (at 278) replied that contraception was not an option due to its many 'side-effects, the full extent of which are not known at the present time'. Moreover there was:

> the difficulty that arises because she is violent from time to time in her mood swing and the difficulties that may arise from effectively *enforcing* over the years that the pill is taken each and every day (ibid.).

Additionally, B was repeatedly described as unlikely to understand the causal connection between intercourse and pregnancy, incapable of forming a long-term adult relationship and devoid of maternal instincts (at 207 and 213):

> ... she has no maternal instincts and is unlikely to develop any. She does not desire children, and if she bore a child she would be unable to care for it.

It is evident that 'desire' here is presented as dependent upon ability to intend to become pregnant. Given that the 'right to procreate' can be understood as the right to obsessive responsibility, it is quite interesting to throw back at the judge his words: 'I do not intend responsibility for B, and if I produce judgement I am unable to accept responsibility for it.' There was more:

> By depriving her of what ... [is] described as the 'basic human right', i.e. the right of woman to reproduce one is in effect depriving her of *nothing* because *she will never desire the 'basic human right to reproduce'* and indeed, on the facts of the case, [to let her become pregnant] would be positively harmful for her (at 213; my emphasis).

In a way, therefore, the judgements held B 'responsible' for her own predicament: she was being 'outside' the realm of responsibility for another being. She was thus held to be an 'irresponsible' being, unable to form relationships and devoid of maternal 'instinct'. Moreover, the judges pathologised the potential exposure to unintended impregnation of this inherently 'irresponsible', care-less being-for-itself, that was B. Hence, it was thought likely that she would be 'terrified, distressed and extremely violent during labour'. In short, reproduction could be 'positively harmful' for *her* and, 'therefore', sterilisation would be 'therapeutically necessary' and in line with B's 'best interests'. As to the point of law, Lord Hailsham did consider *Re D* but said that the judge there had rightly emphasised the irreversible nature of the operation of sterilisation and the ensuing endangerment of the right to reproduce in case the patient's intelligence increases. In consequence, he said, this right was *only* valid when 'reproduction was the result of informed choice', which B clearly lacked (at 213). Lords Bridge and Oliver also linked the existence of such right to reproduce with the mother's capacity to make an informed choice (respectively at 204, 219). Relying on the difference of facts between the two cases to support his view (basically the diagnoses and prognoses of actual and future intelligence), Lord Hailsham concluded that, while *Re D* had been correctly decided, '[t]o talk of the 'basic right' to reproduce of an individual who is not capable of knowing the causal connection between intercourse and childbirth, the nature of pregnancy, what is involved in delivery, and who was unable to form maternal instincts or to care for a child, appears to me wholly to part company with reality' (ibid.).

But of course the judge's determination not to part company with 'reality' says more about himself than about B. Indeed, although the formulation 'devoid of maternal instincts' remains an unsafe attribution to the ward, it makes perfect sense as a self-description of judicial *indifference*. If the (obliquely) generic term maternal 'instinct' is to retain a specific relationship with the human being it is in connoting the *involuntariness* of parental love as responsibility. To the injury of B's incapacity is thus added the insult of accusing her of being, effectively, less than a mammalian organism with inherent 'instincts'. To her incapacity to manifest her desire to be-for-another in a way that others find intelligible, was added the extra accusation of being unable 'to form' long-lasting relationships. In summary, in *Re B* the non-sense of B's situation was appropriated as *legal* nonsense.   Irresponsibly and hypocritically, the legal judgment reserved all emphasis for (and interest in) B the 'imbecile', described as being physically and mentally unable to have a 'harmless' childbirth.

The urgent question is, how was such a development at all possible?   Already in *Re D* - and that makes the latter a much less satisfactory judgment than it first appeared - the judge had hidden her subjective responsibility for her 'compassionate' decision to defend a woman's right to responsibility in the form of right to procreation as being independent of the relative presence/absence of autonomy and agency. It is sad but not surprising that D's judge was thus shown to be blind to how both the patient in question and the judge herself are subjects of humanity in bearing a complex right to responsibility which is both a burden and a condition of freedom and individuation. The otherwise liberal *Re D* falsely substituted calculation for obsession: weighing the patient's 'terror' and 'distress' during labour against the detrimental effects that sterilisation would have on the patient.   As such, *Re D* is a judgment which gave birth to new law but refused to 'accept parenthood'.

Re D and *Re B* are ultimately characterised by irresponsibility towards the non-sensical suffering which prevents an incompetent woman *intending* to become responsible-for-another. In the 'calculus of risks' of the sterilisation and pregnancy to the woman's health and/or psychological well-being there is no space for addressing the absurdity of the situation.[8] In *Re D* the judge's determination to present the decision as if the result of a syllogism or choice led her to state that 'apart from the irreversible nature of the operation, [the consequences to the patient] were likely to be minimal' (at 212). Little effort is needed to demonstrate the arbitrariness of the above 'balancing' operation.[9] If indeed being pregnant is originally a state of being responsible for another *despite* one's self, then what we call the 'right to procreate' - the most typical instance of transcending one's self by being responsible for another, which Lévinas brilliantly calls the most fundamental human right - may be *forfeited* to any set of other pressing considerations. For example, given the mother's inability to care for her new baby, the interests of those who will necessarily find themselves *in loco parentis* must be taken into account. Some-*one*-else must help the incompetent become a mother (or else assume responsibility for her sterilisation) without absolving themselves from responsibility due to 'necessity'. Beyond this forfeiture, it cannot logically be said that the right to responsibility exists only in so far as its bearer is 'capable of appreciating its significance'. Yet, unfortunately, this is precisely the misconception in *Re D,* which resulted in a miscarriage in *Re B.*

In the aftermath of these two cases the *only* right to procreation recognised in English law is, as Grubb and Pearl have observed, the right to 'choose whether or not to reproduce' (A. Grubb and D. Pearl 1987: 46). De Cruz rightly remarks that in the above decision their Lordships effectively posited the principle that there is no 'basic right to reproduce' unless the potential parent is capable of appreciating its significance (De Cruz 1988: 10-11). I can only agree with De Cruz that this kind of reasoning is 'neither logically sound nor morally tenable' (ibid. 11), if only for the mere fact that a person's inability to appreciate the significance of a particular right does not entitle another to deprive them of that right. 'Indeed', he continues, alluding to the wardship character of the above cases, 'a child's right to be maintained, educated and protected by persons *in loco parentis* does not derive from that child's appreciation of that right but from the existence of that parental duty' (ibid.). M. D. A. Freeman asks whether the court's position in *Re B* is meant to be the judicial criterion for the exercise of all rights, or exceptionally for the right to reproduce, noting that if it applies to rights in general, it 'would have very

---

[8] For how the conceptualisation of health transforms the absurd into an *enigma* see Hans-Georg Gadamer 1996, espec. chap. 2, 'Apologia for the Art of Healing', 31-43.

[9] No natural labour is stress- and pain-free. Thus one could subvert the judge's statement - and thus his claim that the patient's harmful labour was his primary concern - by saying that apart from the 'irreversible nature' of childbirth a caesarian section would be just as intrusive and equally harmful as sterilisation. One could be forgiven for thinking that the judge considered childbirth as easy as his defense of the rights of incompetents. Further, the judge overlooked the evidence that at the time Jeanette was capable of playing with dolls and therefore could have 'understood', according to the new test of incompetence that I explained in Chapter 2, a simple straightforward explanation of how babies are born and how it was proposed that she should not have any.

strange consequences indeed' (Freeman ed. 1988: 62). Finally, in *Law and Medical Ethics* J. K. Mason and R. A. McCall Smith attempt a defence of the decision in *Re B* which I think is only partly useful. They rightly claim that the resolution of the 'dilemma regarding the right to reproduce cannot be limited and impersonalised' to the single aspect of giving birth but must include an element of aftercare (Mason and McCall Smith 1994: 88). Since some mentally handicapped women are unable to provide this, the recognition of this right then becomes dependent upon the extent of their ability to fulfil this role. In my view, as far as this statement provides for a critique of the individualistic conception of rights it is not at odds with my understanding of the right to reproduce as 'the right to be responsible'. Indeed the mother's responsibility for the foetus as 'the stranger within' cannot possibly be exhausted by the physical and emotional labour of giving birth. In fact with the cutting of the umbilical cord responsibility is only transformed. I must, however, strongly disagree with the view that the right to reproduce depends upon an ability to care for the infant following birth. For it is always unacceptable to assume the irresponsibility (and therefore the in-humanity) of another to the effect of forfeiting the exercise of their rights. And it is even more unacceptable when forfeiting effectively becomes *foreclosing* such exercise under the pretence that rights need to be recognised only when their bearer is 'capable' of appreciating their full significance. In such cases the only safe approach is either to balance competing rights or act in the direction of preventing a case of 'abuse of rights'. With regard to maternity this holds true be it in connection with a mentally competent mother's right not to reproduce or a mentally incompetent prospective mother's right to do so. In short, the ability to provide care after birth must be considered to be merely of demonstrative value to the right to become pregnant which exists even when this ability is missing.

The perspective of Mason and McCall reflects an attitude deeply embedded in much jurisprudence. This sets up a 'dilemma' between 'rights'-holders and the principle of welfare and concern for the more vulnerable, then attempts to resolve the 'dilemma' by sponsoring a choice in one or other direction. We can think, for instance, of the divide between supporters of children's 'adult-like' rights, and those who claim the parental right to treat children as 'children', i.e. as dependant non-adults. In today's liberal climate there is no single criterion for differentiating between adults and their 'other', and even in law, the juridical 'age-status' is no longer considered an appropriate criterion for differentiating between 'subjects of rights' and 'objects of concern'. These circumstances should not alarm supporters on either side of the 'children's welfare comes first' and 'justice for children' opposition, simply because they demonstrate how the recognition of children's rights *presupposes* a parental-type concern towards them. Coming back to the issue of the incompetent adult's right to procreation, we could re-formulate it as the fundamental right to expose oneself to the potentiality of relating to another being as neither fully autonomous nor fully dependent.

III
Affective 'sincerity'

James Boyd-White's approach to 'law as literature' and to 'justice as imagination' is relevant here (Boyd-White 1985, 1990). Boyd-White examines 'law' as a 'system of language' in which claims of meaning are made, reasons are provided and, in short, facts are converted into law. The judging subject is not seen as entirely theoretical or totally formed by the language and knowledge he or she inhabits; instead, subjectivity as field of experience, affectivity and emotion, is wider than what it signifies from within particular languages like the language of law. The problem with legal language is one of 'defective expressiveness'. In order to understand issues of justice in medical litigation, he argues, we have to begin by interrogating the capacity of the 'language of the law' to express the emotions which qualify the responsibility to care. As it happens the language of law - that of autonomy and formal equality - is not adequate to express the impact of human suffering on the law judge who witnesses it. Boyd-White's theory of legal imagination and 'justice as translation' has evolved from his previous commentaries on judicial decisions on the end(ing) of life of patients in *The Legal Imagination* (1985: 71-108). There he read closely a series of judicial judgments, and, by demonstrating the tension between facts and law, narrative and theory, he found that the legal language which lawyers inherit as acceptable in legal proceedings is an 'incomplete system of expression'. Point by point he showed how the judges who are faced with extreme forms of human suffering are barred by their own professional language from expressing their actual experience of and feeling towards patients and those burdened with care-duties.

However, legal discourse is also constantly interrupted and contradicted by that which it strives to leave out: emotional and other aspects of the judges' overall experience of the matter which do not fit the formal logic of 'applying the law'. Boyd-White ascribes this phenomenon to the 'force of narrative' as a 'pressure towards the inexpressible' which 'takes a life of its own'. The interruptions and inherent contradictions that Boyd-White detects are no different from what more traditional critics of the law have called evidence of 'absurdity' and 'legal fantasy'. In my first chapter we saw examples of these. But with what ethical and justificatory *sense* does Boyd-White's theory of 'justice as interpretation' wish to tackle these 'absurdities'? According to his general premises, legal judgments, as all acts of language, are actions in the world, not just in our minds. From this perspective of decisions as 'speech acts', Boyd-White thus calls us to look through the theory that sustains so-called 'objective' and 'neutral' medico-legal judgment in order to re-discover the ethical and political sense of the personal judgement that lies beneath. In short, Boyd-White is interested in *exposing* the subjectivism of medical legal judgement. The 'justice' of a decision does not lie in its substantive content but in the recognition by the decision-maker of the political and ethical character of his decision in relation to others. Justice becomes a matter of the *sincerity* with which the judge 'expresses' his intentions.[10] In order to be sincere the lawyer must first acknowledge the limits of institutional legal language. Not all his intentions towards the judged can be expressed by use of legal language (for example emotional intentions). So to be 'expressive' the judgment must recognise both the 'lawyer' and the 'non-lawyer' that speak it. The way to achieve this is to render explicit the so-called 'narrative tension' in the legal judgment. This is a tension between theory and facts, knowledge and emotions. The lawyer must 'look elsewhere', beyond legal language, for the means of 'control of the narrative'.

James Boyd-White's 'narrative tension' does not yet account for the passivity of the medical lawyer *qua* human 'witness of absurd suffering'. In the so-called 'sincere' legal talk whereby the lawyer says more than he states, there is no provision for the speechlessness a subject may experience before unimaginable and utterly absurd human suffering. Boyd-White's theory continues, it seems, a tradition of assuming the potential triumph of human consciousness over suffering. By contrast, Lévinas helps us trace the obsessive part of the medico-legal judgment. In so far as the delirium in a judgment corresponds to an obsession directed towards the other as the other 'for me' and my responsibility, the judicial subject of consciousness is both 'bound-hostage' *and* 'radically free' to engage its other as 'the only one that matters', and as the one 'for *me*' and my responsibility. The self is ethically free to approach the other obsessively (as 'the' one) and in disinterestedness in the name of responsibility. The fact that the other suffers 'absurdly' and 'for nothing' liberates me to approach him or her *anarchically* - without need to refer to any 'authority' other than *my* desire for a unique other who calls out to *me*. However, I argue, in so far as the 'delirium' of the judgment is absorbed into a principle of absurdity (as in Boyd-White's 'insincere' medico-legal judgment), or even 'mastered' though 'techniques of narrative control', absurdity is *appropriated* by the witness of suffering. Thus the ethical sense of the judging self's encounter with the non-sense and absurdity, to which the other human's suffering points, is lost. This, of course, happens more evidently in so far as a medico-legal judgment is presented as if an 'impersonal' or 'objective' judgment'; but also, I argue, where the 'subjective' element in judgement is acknowledged, not as expression of aimless and obsessive concern for an absurd suffering, but as 'confession' by the judge of his own subjectivity's 'secrets' and 'traumas'; and also where, as in Boyd White's theory, the judge is thought to be capable of absolving himself of responsibility for absurdity by

---

[10]James Boyd-White's view of 'sincerity' is very much like that of 'naivité' in phenomenology. In the latter the subject is capable of exposing its intentions by 'bracketing' all its categories. However, in this sense, sincerity is still an attribute of intentionality. By contrast the Greek word for 'sincerity' shows more the *counter-intentional* aspect: *eilikrineia* is to suffer exposure (from *eili*: light and *krinein*: to judge or to torture, i.e. to be judged or tortured by the light).

acknowledging, sincerely, the limits of his discourse to express this responsibility. In either case a false 'truth' takes the place of the anarchy and non-sense of the being-for-the-other, in a way that allows us to talk of 'appropriation' of absurdity by the objective judgment or the subjective judgement (spelled with and without the extra 'e', respectively, to point to the subject behind the legal decision).

What, then, is the sense of the medico-legal judgment beyond its subjective/objective meaning where non-sense is appropriated, and beyond Boyd-White's 'sincerity' over the limits of the legal?[11] The anarchy of the 'for-the-other', where it is impossible to differentiate between me and my other, is replaced by the methodological authority of a collective 'way' of knowing (objectivity) and/or it reverts to the substantive intimity and internal dialogue of the soul with itself, in being-for-itself (subjectivity). However, Lévinas calls on us to resist the belief that the ultimate secret of subjectivity lies 'only' in the intimity of the soul's dialogue with itself, or that it is 'only' 'constructed' in the public sphere. The equation between universality and individuation is never solved; it is better addressed by Lévinas' model, where, paradoxically, the individual is said to be passively 'cast in the role' of responsible being *albeit* this is a 'role' which belongs to the human being as of right - as its first right. The individual has to claim its right to serve the other.

Nevertheless, it remains true that the legal judgment often specifically defers to established knowledge and ways of looking at the world, and so obscures the intimate link between the subjectivity of the judge and the judgment he or she makes, so as to maintain the internal coherence of the 'system' of law as a distinctive, closed interiority of meaning. This is especially obvious in cases dealing with death and 'absurd' human suffering, where there is an abundance of circular interpretations of legal doctrine. These are not errors or distortions. On the contrary they show that at the most fundamental level the very existence of sovereign legal judgment entails an irresponsible 'appropriation' of the absurdity of the death and suffering of the other human, as well as an exploitation of the other's passive situation. For instance the doctrine of 'sanctity of life' operates today more like a 'principle of absurdity' authorising a certain moral indifference. Even beyond so-called 'hard' medical law cases, there are many interesting doctrinal anomalies and recurring ambiguities in relation even to the most 'mundane' legalistic issues surrounding responsibility for 'ordinary' patients. Ideally, because of the subject-matter *medical law* cases should be given a privileged position in the study of the ethics of law and jurisprudence. They involve decisions which challenge legal determinism on matters which - in the

---

[11]To pose this specific question is also, by implication, to question Kant's scepticism which Boyd-White extends to language. I mean that Boyd-White seems to affirm the limits of legal knowledge and the creative possibilities resulting from an acknowledgment of these limits, as if this encapsulated the ethical sense of being affected by my other's 'useless' suffering.

most explicit of ways - invite the re-thinking of the meaning of political and civil society; they point towards the surprise of the 'disinterested' but emotionally engaged community between beings who have nothing in common - not even an ontology - but who are in each other's service. Yet unfortunately, legal doctrine is at present remarkably repetitious.

IV
The exceptionalisation of the
doctor-patient relationship in medical law

In general, the doctor-patient relationship occupies an ambiguous area in the modern western world. On the one hand the patients' expectations and the medical profession's Hippocratic allusion to a sacred past shroud it with the mantle of an intimate and highly ethical relationship.[12] This partially explains why, unlike all other transactions, it is not ruled by ordinary law. On the other hand, we go in the opposite direction when we account for the way in which this relationship of power is 'materialised' today (as in the impersonal, technological environment of modern hospitals). It is, we hear, loaded with a 'normalising' function that complements the state's political means of control of inter-subjectivity with 'technologies of self governance' that penetrate deeply into the individual body. This ambivalence between the two opposite accounts of the clinical affair appears at present irreconcilable. The legal view is no less ambivalent. In England, Common law's ambiguity towards the doctor-patient relationship goes in tandem with a persistent 'exceptionalisation' of responsibilities owed to patients, under obscure policy considerations and by means of rather unhappy legal formulations. Let me give a few examples. Strict medical liability is not accepted either in England or in North America. The English approach is solely contractual and generally seen as the one with the lowest standards of medical responsibility (Kennedy and Grubb 1994: Introduction).

However, for the English judge, the contract between sufferer and doctor is also a very 'special' one.[13] By way of comparison, Canadian courts, usually seen as passing quite innovative medical law judgments, recognise the relationship to

---

[12]On this matter see Pellegrino *et al.*, eds. 1991, and Ehrenreich 1978, Komesaroff ed. 1995.

[13]'[there is] no comparison to be made between the relationship of doctor and patient with that of solicitor and client, trustee and cestui qui trust or the other relationships treated in equity as of a fiduciary chararacter. *Nevertheless*, the relationship remains a very *special* one, the patient putting his life in the doctor's hands' (per Lord Scarman in *Sidaway v. Board of Governors of the Bethlem Royal Hospital* [1985] AC 871 [1985] 1 All E.R. 643) as cited by Kennedy and Grubb 1994: 175; my emphasis.

be of a fiduciary character. However, again, a very particular sense is attributed which does not apply to other such relationships of trust. Thus, the higher responsibility which that trust normally entails is mitigated, especially in the case of the doctor, by the concurrent use of the so-called 'reasonable patient' test as well as by the existence of a special defence called 'therapeutic privilege'.[14] The former is easily understood whilst the latter is a defence that can be claimed by doctors who refused to disclose 'distressing' facts to their patient. It is important to note that it extends, not to 'distress' in general, but to distress that is likely to have negative effects on the patient's treatment, causing him/her to feel 'resigned' and thus less collaborative with the physician. Focusing on English law, I relate this ambivalence to the development of case law which admittedly sets very low standards for medical responsibility *without*, however, changing the basic legal premises. For even under such low standards judges go to great lengths in order to desist from protecting patients in a way that pits them against their doctors. Under these circumstances there is a sense that there has been an abandonment of the rule of law in the field of medical malpractice, and a sense that medical paternalism is judicially endorsed. The patient's consent appears merely a subordinate aspect of the therapeutic process. The plaintiff-patient's basic human right of self-determination may be defeated by the purely medical decision of his doctor, as endorsed by the courts.[15]

In other words, both in the clinic and in court, the patient is accustomed to being considered as a pawn on the chessboard of medical circumstance, and brings himself more often to suffer the therapy than to take part in it. One has many other reasons to complain of abandonment of the 'rule of law' in this area, as, for example, the well-known *Bolam* principle whereby the law lays down the duty of care but leaves the standards of care to medicine. There are also the issues of the scope of the patient's 'informed' consent of which I shall speak later. For now, let me concentrate on the unjustified policy of declaring the doctor-patient relationship 'special' and exceptional; in the event this happens in order to derail medical law cases from the path of litigation. In this regard the judges often speak of the 'necessity' of preventing a 'flood of medical litigation' and of stopping the phenomenon of 'defensive medicine' from spilling over from the other side of the Atlantic. Overall, the message English judges prefer to send is that 'informal resolution' and out-of-court settlement and negotiation are preferable to litigation

---

[14] See Kennedy and Grubb 1994: 200. 'It must now only be a matter of time before English law adopts the "reasonable patient" test.'

[15] The three most important such instances relate to: (a) public health or other prevailing public interest (the law imposes a duty to receive treatment upon persons suffering from certain communicable and venereal diseases, but also prisoners and the inmates of mental hospitals may be compelled to submit to certain medical procedures; examples include prisoners on hunger strikes who may be lawfully force-fed, whilst 'mental prisoners' may be forcibly sterilised); (b) cases of attempted suicide; and (c) emergencies.

with regard to doctor-patient disputes; at least in Britain, this message has now been officially endorsed by the state and the medical associations. However, this 'anti-legalistic' policy of lawyers, especially with regard to complaints by patients, only seemingly serves public interest. The fear of a 'flood of medical litigation' may appear understandable in the context of a state like Britain which still concentrates considerable resources in a national health system, but it is in fact 'unsubstantiated' (Cabe *et al.*, eds. 1994: 46-64).[16] In fact there is a danger that the emphatic mention of the problem of 'defensive medicine' will obscure more relevant considerations.[17] Finally, even if the English courts' anti-litigation policy in relation to medical suits is underlined by considerations of 'access to justice', it would appear not to have learned anything from the shortcomings of the informalist movement a decade earlier.[18]

The ambiguity in the judicial perception of the doctor-patient relationship leads to taxonomic ambivalence and relates to the 'arrested' development of legal doctrine in this area - in spite of the relative increase in suits in medical litigation. I submit that the development of medico-legal doctrine is arrested, among other reasons, by an indifference to the peculiar 'subject-matter' of the doctor-patient relationship, i.e. pure, human suffering on the part of those who have been trained to calculate the representable and quantifiable. 'Medical law' was initially seen as a mere subset of liability laws but has gradually been recognised as subject to principles of 'human rights' law. This change in perception is often associated, with good reason, with the progress of medical technology. The phenomenon, however, is not, as some people have it, due to the capacity of 'extraordinary' technology to create 'new' situations with moral problems that supposedly humanity had never faced before (such as, for example, the 'vegetating' patient). Rather, the emergence of technology which is capable of intervening in the life of the unique human being, not only from the cradle (where its unicity is manifested externally) but even prior to its conception, simply makes more apparent the

---

[16]More litigation does not mean more successful claims; nor is there any proof that patients who are losing patience with their doctors are more patient with the delays and expenses of the legal system.

[17]For instance, it may be claimed to be the main reason behind the significant decline in natural births in the USA. Indeed caesarians are less likely to be followed by complications and so are legally 'safer' options for litigation-weary doctors. Yet the appeal of complication-free caesarians can be explained in a number of different ways other than that they are less risky.

[18] See later, my Chapter 6. Here, it suffices to say that outside the formal court system there is no vacuum of justice that tribunals can fill; bargaining and negotiation between patients and doctors can only be heavily endowed with court-like adjudicative reasoning and only be preamble to more serious legal measures. Nor are mediation and settlement significantly less bureaucratic and costly ways of resolving medical disputes. By its very nature the field of medical complaints management and resolution is open to the need for 'expert' and costly advice.

heteronomous nature of the constitution of life and subjectivity. In such a context, thankfully, it has become more difficult for medical law to conceal the radical passivity of the legal subject too.

For me, the noted ambiguity in the way the doctor-patient relationship is seen indicates more than an 'accidental' impact of medical technology on law. First and foremost, I submit, it is the *legal* technologies of self which prevent a lawyer from doing justice to all that is involved in the doctor-patient relationship, as well as in the relationship between the law judge himself and each of the disputants. The legal emphasis on autonomy and agency forecloses the discussion of matters of medical/legal ethics on the grounds of ethical subjectivity. Ethical subjectivity is always 'free as well as bound', in situations of so-called 'tragic dilemma' and 'hard choice', to respond with one-way acts of disinterested engagement. The other is then obsessively approached as 'otherwise than being/not-being' and as unique - not in the sense of subjective or objective difference but as the only human among many that matters for *me*. Normally, therefore, the judging subject is free to assert its right in being responsible for the other as 'its' only other. This right to personal responsibility must be seen as 'the first human right' rather than be obscured by the legal sense of proximity and intentional assumption of responsibility. None of this is directly expressible at present in medical law.

V
The scene of irresponsibility for suffering: scientific medicine

I showed in Chapter 1 how the figure of the judge, presented as if an unemotional consciousness, is central to the belief that modern law lives on as a self-referential system of positive rules and as instances of impersonal, 'formal' adjudication on inter-subjective harm. What I mean by the judge who has been abstracted from exposure to 'affectivity beyond experience' (specifically in the form of encountering the judged-other as subject to unintelligible suffering) has already been made clear on different occasions in the preceding chapters: he or she is only an autonomous agent of law, an incorrigible calculator of harm and benefit, rights and interests. Supposedly incapable of transcending his or her self-same identity and agency, he or she cannot be moved by the other's incomparable, absurd suffering. What is obliterated is the counter-intentional subjectivity of the judge as subject to upsetting emotions and contradictory logic. The '*ex officio*' judge of suffering is 'banned' from being affected excessively by another's suffering. Perhaps the same can now be said of modern scientific medicine.

Epistemologists may claim that medicine, like positive law, could not have developed as a science without foreclosing in the process the subjectivity of both doctor and patient. Indeed, every 'separate' scientific field is constituted necessarily through an original act of isolating its proper empirical 'object'.

Retroactively, this 'object' gives each science its anchorage in a world of obscure and fluctuating reality, but also its coherence, its orientation, its methods. But for this process to succeed a second condition must be met. The subjectivity of the scientist (for example the scientific doctor) must not count, or at least, must intervene as insignificantly as possible, in the obtaining of results (therapy). Also, the object of scientific endeavour (for example the patient) must *not* be human subjectivity, i.e. the person of the patient, but merely one or another of its effects, e.g. somatic or psychological benefit. However, I want to challenge the view that specifically medical progress is incompatible with being-for-the-other, and argue that without the vocations of obsessive compassion, 'scientific', 'professional' medicine is missing orientation. This is important for our understanding of a doctor's responsibilities for its counter-intentional actions and decisions upon another's suffering - i.e. those which the doctor could not have intended. Thankfully modern medicine successfully disengaged itself from the dogmatism it had inherited from Aristotle and from the often irrational empiricism of the 'barber-doctors'.[19] To be sure, this process involved what Lévi-Strauss has called *la pensée de l'ingénieur,* which is founded, among other things, on the recourse to measured experience. However I argue that this kind of thought was only the key to the *efficacy* of technical medical progress (pharmacological or other), and was *not,* as it may appear, a *sufficient* condition for the enormous progress that has been achieved by scientific medicine, which I claim, lies in medicine's call, *firstly,* to provide relief to the subject of 'useless' and 'absurd' suffering, and only *secondly* to be concerned with experiencing and understanding disease.

I accept that the constitutive 'object' of modern scientific medicine was the physiology and biology of the human body, and, moreover, that the founding act of scientific medicine implicated an 'exclusion' (perhaps an indifference) towards the subjectivity of either doctor or patient. This kind of opinion, however, refers to the eviction of subjectivity as 'content' or 'mode of being' of the subject of consciousness. It does not describe the relation between subjects of suffering as extreme passivity and unintentional responsibility for this absurd passivity. It is not enough to explain the epistemic 'necessity' that there can be no place for subjectivity 'as content' in modern therapy. There is also, in modern medicine, an ignorance of its 'purpose' to exist 'for nothing', as having no higher reference than every patient's relief. I claim that the suppression of the individual vocation of compassion for absurd human suffering, is a particularly unnecessary 'evil' among modern care-professionals, but evident in the institutionalised hierarchisation of the tasks of both nurses and doctors.

Perhaps, however, scientific progress in medicine is not necessarily incompatible with subjectivity in the ethical sense. Medicine is ineluctably connected to individuated subjectivity as the 'emotional witness' of suffering.

---

[19]For a discussion of Aristotle's views see Hans-Georg Gadamer 1996, espec. chap. 2, 'Apologia for the Art of Healing': 31-43.

Medicine responds to absurd suffering primarily with obsessive offering of succour and relief. Succour is wider than 'cure'. It is provided by means of actions which are more 'patient' and 'gratuitous' than curative ones, although they appear more 'urgent' in temporal terms. The rationalisation and systematisation of medical knowledge is said to require an 'objective' and detached approach to human suffering, most graphically in the course of scientific experimentation. Beyond the horizons of curable/incurable organic conditions the doctor is at once bound and free to provide assistance and relief of suffering. This points to the fact that strength and freedom are inherent in the helplessness of the witness of the absurdity which is human suffering. Non-therapeutic provision of relief is not a negligible aspect in the constitution of medicine although it has been the subject of indifference in the history of modern scientific medicine. Therefore, beyond the 'social' sense we make of the doctor-patient association, especially in terms of its 'function' as institutionalised field of regulation and control, it is worth studying the non-sense of this relationship.

How, then, to do justice to the expectations that patients cannot be asked to give up, of intimate, individualised attention to their needs and desires? How not to overlook the existential and ethical pressures on medical professionals who, contrary to popular belief, never cease to be amazed and shocked by the scandal of human suffering? I submit that the subjective 'disinterest' that medical scientific progress requires from the doctor should not be confused with, nor expected to manifest itself as inertia and lack of affectivity beyond experience, or as active achievement of 'emotional indifference'. Even when it is said that a doctor examines a terminal case 'only' in order to gather knowledge for the benefit of future 'similar' patients, he or she is inescapably responding to the demand for succour by the unique patient. Medical progress is not the result of the accumulation of knowledge on the basis of experience of suffering. Technical progress and advances in knowledge are sustained by, but *not* created by, the resolve and discipline of doctors, who often have to rein in their insatiable appetite for compassion towards the suffering of patients whose death or deterioration cannot be averted. Is it, therefore, safe to presume that ceasing to 'care' mindlessly for my other's absurd suffering is a *sine qua non* for responsible professional conduct, thus equating responsible with sober, unemotional conduct? In terminal cases, doctors are told in their schools, they must persist with their focus on 'cure' instead of relief. It is thus that the patient becomes a 'case' and an object of experimentation for the sake of future 'similar' patients and the social body. As such, the 'suffering other' ceases to be unique and becomes 'different' from but equal to others. However, I argue, the scientific medical progress which is solely justified in terms of calculation and utilitarianism and refuses to invest in relief 'for nothing' is *disorientated* progress.

Today's revival of 'traditional' healing practices, precisely at the moment when scientific medicine has delivered and continues to deliver on its promises - may indicate something more than a force 'complementary' to the scientific medicine which reinforces medical institutional 'dominance' of society in our times.[20] We can be sure of only one thing, namely, that sufferers will always seek help from anyone who professes to alleviate suffering.[21] In this connection, the predominant medico-academic models of the doctor-patient relationship and of the aim of treatment, from the nineteenth through the twentieth century, have repeatedly suppressed the significance of the demand for succour and the urge to alleviate suffering in favour of an interest in the patient as therapeutic 'object'. In medical history the two predominant models are referred to respectively as 'scientific-nihilism' and the 'patient-centred movement'. In 1841 the Viennese academic Joseph Dietl, a pupil of the famous physician Josef Skoda, was already defining the task of medicine as not at all healing, but 'research into scientific mechanisms' (*Cambridge History of Medicine* 1996: 138). Bernhard Naunyun, who later became a professor of internal medicine in Germany, remembered of his professors in Berlin in the 1860s that:

> They knew that the curing part of medicine rested upon the discipline's scientific basis, and that the physician's compulsion to heal [*Drang zum Heilen*] had to be reined in (CHM: 142).

These two voices express the justifiable scepticism that had descended upon doctors in the second part of the nineteenth century, prior to the onset of the great pharmacological revolution. Doctors were exasperated by the indiscriminate use of ineffective and sometimes dangerous drugs by practitioners who would promise their patients an easy 'cure'. Their scepticism about the possibilities of drug treatment in general was then logically and ethically justified. Yet only good followed: effort and resources ceased being directed primarily towards 'heroic' medical practices, and pharmacological research produced the first antibiotics.

---

[20]Literature, particularly sociological literature, is ever increasing on the subject of medicine as an institution of control and power. Apart from Michel Foucault's own work (Foucault 1971, 1973, 1974, 1979, 1980, 1987, 1988) indicative is the most extensive work by B. S. Turner: 1980, 1981, 1985, 1987, 1992, 1995.

[21]Early doctors would prescribe laxatives and other dubious concoctions, and at times dangerous infusions ; a whole generation of opiate addicts owed their addiction to those 'charlatans'. Love of the patient's money or gratitude, above the recognition that the truly scientific physician can expect for the cures he or she effects, can 'absorb' much more of the caring subject's 'insatiable compassion'; thus, the quack feels much freer to engage in risky, one-way actions of relief. The appeal of quacks lay in their understanding of the aim of medicine as being primarily palliation and comfort, rather than cure. These two 'aims' (or rather demands) of treatment, I argue, constitute the diachronic and pre-original call to medicine, including today's scientific medicine. And it is in this light that I understand today's dissatisfaction with scientific medicine - at the same time that science has conferred success over much of the vast range of diseases that plague humanity! Scientific doctors today suffer the effects of the delimitation of the form and content of the compassion they are free to have as ethical subjectivities.

However, the phenomenon of scepticism soon gave rise to an attitude aptly described as 'therapeutic nihilism', and it is interesting to study why. Nihilism is an attempt to harness self-interested doctor-heroics in attempting to cure where that was futile or even dangerous for the patient. Yet it was also a denial of the 'insatiable desire' to provide relief for incurable and, so, 'useless' suffering. Consider the nihilist view as to what constitutes the 'real' function of medicine:

> In the second half of the nineteenth century the nihilists ruled the roost in academic medicine, teaching generations of medical students...that physicians could do relatively little to cure disease (although they could relieve suffering with opium), and, *by implication*, that the real function of medicine was to accumulate scientific information about the human body rather than to heal (ibid. 138; my emphasis).

From a nihilistic perspective relief of pain in itself was perhaps a 'morally good' act, but it was not one which was rightly at the top of a physician's mind (it was of little scientific interest): hence, it was left to 'secondary' staff. Nurses - and the first anaesthetists - were to be regarded as little more than technical aides. The message was that the difference between the 'right' (nihilistically trained) physician and the wrong one (charlatan) was that although both wanted to and could relieve useless suffering, only the former would abandon palliation unless it accompanied or contributed to proper scientific work. In other words, there is a banishment or marginalisation of the action of relief which is scientifically 'useless' and only of 'secondary' social value as compared to the prevention and cure of common disease. It is my argument that this 'message' is echoed in the legal profession', and that it still resonates in the form of suspension of the rule of law and the disrespect for human rights in the doctor-patient relationship.

'Patient-centred' medical practice followed 'therapeutic nihilism'. It related to a 'consumerist' approach to patient self-determination, and still characterises, in particular, American medical law.[22] The movement is described in the *Cambridge History of Medicine* as a 'backlash' against nihilism and a return to earlier romantic medicine (CHM: 142). There I read that the Viennese Professor of Medicine Hermann Nothnagel was fond of quoting a saying from a romantic figure of German medicine, Christoph Wilhelm Hufeland, to the effect that 'only a truly moral person can become a physician in the truest sense of the term'. However, it can be argued that the patient-as-a-person doctrine that Nothnagel espoused was far more engaged with the nihilists than the word 'backlash'

---

[22]It ran through primary care from the 1880s until the second world war. In Vienna, Hermann Nothnagel, professor of medicine after 1882, was one of the first to embrace the new attitude. As he said in his inaugural lecture, 'I repeat once again, medicine is about treating sick people and not diseases'. He was known to be a 'friend of the patient', emphasising the importance of history-taking in the consultation - a key theme in the movement as a whole, because in taking a long and careful history the doctor has the chance to establish emotional rapport with the patient (CHM).

suggests. It was in fact a movement *marked* by nihilism, and only a perverse return to the morality of romantic medicine. Nothnagel advocated seeing the patient as 'a person' and not as 'a case of disease' *only* in so far as it could be argued that the physician's understanding and sympathetic approach was 'in and of itself therapeutic' (CHM: 143). Thus so-called 'patient-centred' medical practice was perhaps a twist in the history of that therapeutic nihilism which had dominated medical schools and effectively banned excessive concern with 'succour' from driving medical progress. In this model, too, as with medical 'paternalism', the doctor is presumed to be unaffectable by absurd, useless suffering, and as radically irresponsible for the other's illness and passivity, and the patient may thereafter be treated as an object. The injunction that doctors must pretend to listen to their patients' stories for the 'patients' therapeutic good' completes the process of de-subjectivisation in the clinical encounter. It turns the doctor into an indifferent ear that listens to everything but what the patient cannot tell - his vulnerability. Doctors were asked to establish a 'rapport', not with a person but with a physical entity.[23] The 'foreclosure' of the subject operated equally amongst those doctors who complemented their therapeutic objective with a psychological one. Suffice it to consider a Dr Daniell Cathell's famous *Doctors' Guide* of 1924:

> It is often very satisfying *to the sick* to be allowed to tell, in their own way, whatever they deem important for you to know. Give a fair, courteous hearing, and, even though Mrs Chatterbox, Mr Borum, and Mrs Lengthy's statements are tedious, do not abruptly cut them short, but endure and listen with respectful attention, *even though you are ready to drop exhausted* (CHM: 145; my emphasis).

Irrespective of how 'satisfying' it is for a sufferer to be 'listened to' as if still an interesting interlocutor although heard as a chatterbox, at a time when his personality is 'under threat', it is certain that the doctor's job becomes easier and his conscience is appeased thereby. If there are still things to be done, he has earned himself a docile patient - if not, at least the patient has 'benefited psychologically' from being heard. Seen through the nihilistic filter therapeutic knowledge increases, as it were, 'in spite' of the expression by the patient of a

---

[23]It is significant that in the process of turning the therapeutic defeats into a triumph for 'right' knowledge and 'good' medical practice there has been remarkably little *proper* scientific development in the field of palliation which is the pharmacological way of addressing useless suffering. Thus at the time when antibiotics were discovered doctors were still giving opiates in the ineffective manner of the early nineteenth century - by mouth. It took an accident to show that opiates had better effect in case of extreme pain when injected rather than swallowed. For similar evidence of neglect closer to our own day, it suffices to say that an entire field of medical research, psychoneuroimmunology - the field that tackles the effects of prolonged mental stress on the body's immune system - has been founded by accident.

therapeutically '*useless*' suffering, i.e. suffering which does not 'offer itself' for knowing but calls for urgent actions and succour. The primacy of palliative care is thus, metonymically, associated exclusively with cases of extremely painful terminal conditions. But even in these cases the task that medicine sets itself is to understand and control the 'sensory excess' of suffering rather than to respond to its 'useless' dimension. Suffering is thus seen as at once 'extreme' and 'exceptional'.

One must be careful not to charge historical accident with the gravity of the essentially unavoidable. What transpires from the brief historiographical points I raised above is that the 'de-subjectification' of the doctor-patient relationship was not the 'inevitable price' paid for the progress of medical science. Rather, it is indicative of a specific attitude of interest in being's essence *coupled* with a certain indifference towards suffering which is seen as extreme, or 'necessary', or insignificant, and towards the ethical proximity as responsibility this suffering entails. The observation that no science can emerge without the act that differentiates or separates off its proper 'object' can now be revisited. To make the point, the meanings of the French verb *se dégager*, as listed by the *Oxford French Dictionary* (2nd ed.), can be used to illustrate how, in relation to the suffering he/she 'witnesses', the modern scientific doctor must indeed *se dégage* - i.e. first, 'disengage' from it, in the sense that he/she must 'separate' or 'sort out' suffering; must, in other words, approach it responsibly and in a disinterested manner, without prejudice, without fear of contamination or anticipation of triumph, and yet with an assertion of an ancient right/moral obligation to 'free' or 'release' the suffering other. However, when *se dégager* is attached to *sa parole* or *sa responsabilité*, it means 'to go back on one's words' and 'to decline responsibility'. In this regard, when the right to responsibility for the 'useless' suffering that oppresses my other is stated, or *said,* then there is a danger that, through lapse of personal responsibility, it cannot have the further meaning: 'to emit', 'to give off'. What is it that could be emitted? That responsibility is also delirious *Saying* directed at the other as *my other*. In sum, the 'right to responsibility' has been claimed by modern medicine in a way which forecloses more than subjectivity as 'psychological content': it forecloses the possibility of the caring subject and of the suffering patient to refer, respectively, the former his/her actions and decisions and the latter his/her passivity, to nothing other than a 'right' to responsibility for what is 'useless' suffering.[24] In the case of modern medicine the attitude of scientific nihilism (not science in itself) represents the first time in history when the medical subject was seen as radically irresponsible

---

[24] This is just as pertinent for a discussion of legal doctrine. For example medical law penalises the patient who had nothing to say about her suffering (as discussed earlier in the case of Ms Northern). In Chapter 4 the case of Ms Sidaway will show that judges disapproved of that patient's failure actively to protect herself against unwanted acts of medical intrusion by asking her doctor a lot of questions.

for useless suffering. Lévinas' view of care is that every human who suffers absurdly must be met by another who will suffer an infinite responsibility in their place. The opposite is true in the doctrine of medical nihilism: therapeutic methodology must be meaningful to the patient, although to the subjectively indifferent doctor it may remain absurd. If medical science now seems 'without human face' it is not because of technical progress, but because it is now almost impossible to conceptualise the kind of proximity that incorporates thematisation, calculation and objectification, as well as the risk of non-sense in the obsession of gratuitous care - care given 'for nothing'. Moreover, the suspension of the rule of law in the area of medical responsibility, which I discussed earlier, indicates a similar sort of loss of faith.

CHAPTER 4

Medico-legal Mysteries

... only a being whose solitude has reached a crispation through suffering, and in relation with death, takes its place on a ground where the relationship with the other becomes possible. The relationship with the other will never be the feat of grasping a possibility (TO: 76).

I
Legal ambivalence towards the doctor-patient relationship

Let me come back to the abeyance of the rule of law in the area of doctor-patient relationships which I examined earlier. It is submitted that the responsibility of doctors who operate without consent, or on the basis of an ineffective consent, is systematically 'de-criminalised', by both American and English courts, for no other reason than a certain judicial reluctance to stigmatise doctors as violent criminals.[1] Indeed, it is a legal mystery why a doctor who operates on a patient without valid consent, albeit in good faith and with no malicious intent, is unlikely to be convicted for the crime or tort of battery or, at least, be found liable in negligence for 'technical assault'. All in all, the criminal conviction of a doctor who operates without consent with an honest intention to 'cure' is at present only a 'theoretical possibility' without good justification (Kennedy and Grubb 1994: 89-90).

In reality, there is responsibility only if the defendant was an impersonator, or, generally, the purpose of bodily intervention was from the start other than medically curative. Cases of successful criminal prosecution are limited to misinformation or lack of consent treatments which took place for money-extortion or sexual gratification. In this way, medical care is legally limited (and so delimited) to that which aims principally and verifiably at *cure* as opposed, for

---

[1]At present 'battery' by a practitioner who intervenes without proper consent by the patient may only be pleaded where there was a *complete* absence of consent, or where consent was obtained by fraud or misrepresentation, or where the treatment actually performed was categorically distinct from that to which consent was given. This cautious formulation, which seems to confuse the tort of battery ... with the separate and distinctive torts of fraud and deceit, represents undoubtedly a judicial reluctance to stigmatize doctors in the same manner as violent criminals.

instance, to forms of care which are motivated, say, by lust or money. From a different point of view, it is worth comparing this legal situation with another, whereby, as is well known, medical intervention for the non-curative purpose of 'compassionate euthanasia', whether with consent or not, is likely to incur a criminal conviction for murder (or, 'in the best of cases', for manslaughter; but this only if the court is satisfied that the doctor was 'provoked' by the patient's horrific situation and therefore had 'diminished responsibility'). It is interesting that compassion which is concerned only with the immediate release of the other from suffering thus constitutes an exception to the judicial policy of 'decriminalising' medical responsibility, alongside money-extortion and lust (although interesting, this observation is perhaps not surprising given that, in the century of fascism, political society accepts that compassion is a form of 'selfish behaviour'; hence it is all the more difficult to claim that *without* obsessive compassion there would be no ethical proximity, and without ethical proximity there can be no responsibility, and therefore no law).

However, let me concentrate on the 'decriminalisation' of medical violence perpetrated with an honest intent to cure and stave off death. Things have not always been this way. Assault, battery and the tort of negligence are in principle distinguishable by the existence or non-existence of 'intent' to act for the purpose of accomplishing a result which the actor knows to be substantially certain; they do *not* require intent to do 'harm', nor evidence of 'hostility'. Thus, in an early twentieth-century American case the judge found that as a matter of law the action of a doctor who operated on the anaesthetised patient's left ear, although only the operation on the right one had been agreed, was 'violent assault'.[2] This clear, albeit legalistic position was abandoned in the course of the next few decades (how this occurred will be explained shortly). To summarise the developments let me cite Allan McCoid's 1957 article 'A Reappraisal of Liability for Unauthorised Medical Treatment':[3]

> What appears to distinguish the case of unauthorised operation ... is the fact that in almost all the cases, the doctor is acting in relative good faith for the benefit of the patient. The traditional assault and battery, on the other hand, involves a defendant who is acting for the most part out of malice or in a manner which is considered as 'anti-social'.

And, a few decades later, in 1981, G. Robertson reassesses things as they stand today:

---

[2] Specifically, it 'amounted at least to a technical assault and battery ... [for it was] a violent assault ... [against the] person's immunity, not a mere pleasantry; and even though no negligence is shown, it was wrongful and unlawful' [per J. Brown in *Mohr v. Williams* (1905)] as cited by Kennedy and Grubb 1994: 90-91.

[3] A. McCoid, 'A Reappraisal of Liability for Unauthorised Medical Treatment' (1957) 41 Minnesota LR 381) as cited in Kennedy and Grubb ibid.

judicial policy appears to be in favour of restricting claims in battery to situations involving deliberate, hostile acts, a situation which most judges would regard as *foreign* to the doctor-patient relationship (Kennedy and Grubb 1994: 91-92; my emphasis).

We are therefore faced with a gradual, but also unaccountable process: there is a certain disengagement of the 'doctor-patient relationship' from hostility and violence; there is also an assertion that the violence that law is concerned with at its most crucial level - i.e. that which is criminally banned - does *not* extend to bodily intrusions for curative purposes, although it may attach to *any* other form of intention. This is presumably because an honestly curative intervention is not seen as 'hostile' or 'anti-social'. Of course, it is not so much that violent acts are 'foreign to the doctor-patient relationship' as that any violence that may be foreign is *either* recognised as 'legitimate/illegitimate', *or else* ignored and thus excepted from the scope of criminal normativity.[4]

There appears to be a polarity: whilst a non-curative compassionate intervention remains legally proscribed, even if it is fully accepted by the patient, it is not criminal for cure-seeking doctors to set aside the patient's autonomy. On the one hand, judges except the intention to cure from criminal law and, crucially for the interpretation of the law, declare it 'inherently non-hostile'; in other words we are told that the relevant actions are found to be lawful and, presumably, 'moral' *because* they are 'inherently non-violent' and, presumably, 'inherently good'. In sum, this attitude constitutes a denial of the 'good violence' of the compassion which underlies all care, and a marginalisation of all care that is not aiming principally at cure. On the other hand, a compassionate and respectful act of euthanasia is most likely to be judged as criminal and compared with self-interested, 'quack-type' deception and even rape.

In this connection it is interesting to remember the two possible defences for compassionate euthanasia. As I mentioned in passing above, one could possibly claim 'loss of mind' and diminished responsibility, i.e. partially excuse oneself by presenting one's exposure to the other's absurd suffering negatively, and, further, by accepting the premise that non-intentional, obsessive, freedom to provide relief 'equates' with lack of responsibility. Second, in cases of illnesses which are known to be terminal, i.e. where cure is improbable, and where, additionally, there is 'extreme' pain, i.e. cases whose incurability 'provokes' the interest of the scientist but 'only' as recognisable symptom and pathology, the perpetrator of compassionate euthanasia can rely on the so-called 'double-effect' principle.[5]

---

[4]This point is demonstrated more in cases concerning sado-masochistic practices between consenting adults, and by the subsequent Law Commission paper where it is suggested that medical intervention be classified, together with boxing (!), as a form of violence which *can* be consented to.

[5]For more see Steinbock and Norcross eds. 1994.

According to the latter it is a defence that, where the death of the patient in question followed the sudden administration of tranquillisers and pain-killers in massive quantities that are known to cause suffocation and heart failure, the doctor who prescribed the drugs had 'primarily' intended to provide relief rather than to kill. The death is declared incidental to this primary, and now suddenly legitimate intention, and so is effectively thought to have been inevitable anyway, due to the terminal nature of the illness. Thus construed, 'compassionate euthanasia' appears a matter of cunning intention and speculation. It is interesting that, in spite of all the anxiety modern judges have in relation to making sure that euthanasia does not become an implicit acceptance of the abhorrent principles of *eugenics*, they have issued doctors with a relative 'license' to kill compassionately, albeit only the incurable, in the form of the principle of 'double effect'.

II
Theoretical ambiguities towards the ethics of care

For some writers the problem with medical law's failure to articulate a proper ethics of medical care lies in the characteristics of the 'justice-perspective' of moral problems of care. In this type of argument 'responsibility' as care and charity is entirely disconnected from responsibility as 'justice'. Supposedly, the principles of justice and judgement, representation, analogy and temporisation, are inherently unable to articulate the ethics of caring; and they cannot relate to the spontaneity and urgency or absolute immediacy of the commitment to care. The reasons for this are the legal emphasis on issues of autonomy, consent, patient self-determination, medical professional integrity and formal equality. What is criticised is that medical law focuses on the question of 'who', of the patient and the doctor, is the ultimate decision-maker and is best equipped to 'know'. I have described this phenomenon above as the result of judicial reluctance to face the 'futile' exposure of the non-sense of suffering, which is 'useless' for a system of law in so far as it results in bringing forth the kind of responsibility which is of no interest to law: that of the ethical subject for its counter-intentional acts, its obsessions 'for nothing'. From my point of view it is theoretically restrictive to argue the separation of the ethics of care from the 'justice-perspective' merely because modern positive law assumes that for every problem involving negligent or unwanted care, the right question to ask is 'who decides' or who 'owns' the decision.

Unfortunately, I argue, this is what feminist psychologist Carol Gilligan did when she proposed that we abandon the 'justice perspective' in medical ethics. Gilligan belongs to a school of thought that proclaims the principles of justice to be incompatible with an ethics of care (Gilligan 1982; Frug 1992: 37-49). Her *In a Different Voice* is based on three research projects involving moral choice.

Using an analysis of the language used by her female research subjects, Gilligan constructed a new model of moral development. This model, which is labelled the 'ethic of care', is mainly associated with women's attitudes towards problems emerging in so-called 'affiliative' relationships.[6] Gilligan contrasts the ethic of care called forth in these relationships with the 'rights-model'[7] which she thinks to be critical in the theory-building studies of such prominent male theorists as Freud, Erik Erikson, Jean Piaget and Lawrence Kohlberg. One may say that Gilligan is limited in concentrating exclusively on women's moral attitudes to care. However, she makes clear that although her empirical research focuses exclusively on women's moral attitudes to care, her intention is to articulate a universal 'feminine' ethic of care, and not to depict the impact of sexual difference on attitudes to care.[8] Thus, her views transcend a narrowly defined politics of feminism. More broadly, they are located within a tradition of civic republicanism, or communitarianism, where the predominant values are of responsibility, connection, selflessness and caring as opposed to the dictates of liberal-individualistic political theories which centre around autonomy, self-actualisation and separation (Frug 1992: 46).

More importantly for my purposes, however, Gilligan has been criticised because her ethics of care only 'applies to dealings with one's intimates' (Whitbeck 1996).[9] It is my argument that this accusation is interesting, if only partly correct, because, wisely, Gilligan fails to identify clearly the form and content of those relationships which she names 'affiliative', and which must be salvaged from the male, decisionist 'justice model'. To the degree, however, that

---

[6]The ethic of care is most fully and persuasively described in the chapter 'Concepts of Self and Morality' which is primarily concerned with the results of Gilligan's abortion decision study (Gilligan 1982: 64-105).

[7]The model of rights is more identified with problems of self-actualisation than relational issues, and with a 'just resolution to moral dilemmas', as determined by objective standards. More than half of the individuals who participated in Gilligan's studies were women. The book reveals that, by contrast, Kohlberg did not include any females in the primary study which led to the formation of his six-stage theory of moral development; Gilligan's book also criticises Freud, Erikson and Piaget for subordinating women and feminine developmental issues in their work.

[8]'The different voice I describe is characterised not by gender but theme. Its association with women is an empirical observation ... highlighting a distinction of two modes of thought ... The choice of a girl whose moral judgments elude existing categories of moral development assessment is meant to highlight the issue of interpretation rather than to exemplify sex differences per se.' Gilligan cited in Frug 1992.

[9]'Ethics of care applies to dealings with one's intimates. Work on the ethics of care is helpful in showing how many moral concerns are inexpressible in terms of rights and obligations alone, but does not provide a framework that is adequate to express the many moral issues raised by [medical] technology that concern responsibilities for the well-being of many anonymous others [as opposed to being responsible only for the individual immediately concerned].' Whitbeck 1996: 42-74.

Whitbeck is correct, Gilligan attempted to locate and/or define a 'type' of ethical proximity which exists, as it were, *separately* from the approach of the 'third' who brings the requirement for justice, comparison, measure and decision. From my perspective, in this way she merely describes the abstractly isolated sociality of 'two people on an island' without concern for the outsider, without 'society'. In this connection, I argue, Gilligan's thesis far from upsets law's ambivalent relationship with the ethics of care, as discussed earlier. If we assume that her idea of the relationship of care is comparable to Lévinas' being-for-each-other, we must also conclude that the latter describes the control over the operations of justice of ethical responsibility in proximity, love and charity with *my* other, whilst the former describes a type of isolated intimacy that abdicates its mission to 'supervise' the strictures of justice. To be sure, Gilligan's theoretical view of relationships of care is an attempt to end the situation whereby, as I explained earlier, problems regarding responsibilities within relationships of care for suffering are 'suspended' by medical law as being *sometimes* suitable for law, and for that matter criminal law (through criminalising 'useless' compassion); whilst *at other times* they are said to be 'too intimate and ethical' to be legally interfered with even for the purposes of relatively inoffensive civil adjudication (as by derailing suits by patients from the path of 'adversarial' litigation).

There is, in all this, a persistent presentation of justice and ethics and of their distinct demands as if they were two corresponding terms which signify, respectively, two separate demands: to be 'just' or fair, and to 'care'. Gilligan presupposes that the sober calculation of demands stemming from associations between additive, inter-changeable individuals who are subjects of rights and obligations has nothing to do with the obsessive desire to care for one's suffering other as the only one that matters, as the unique subject of incomparable and utterly unjustifiable or absurd suffering. However, Gilligan also takes a wise step back, by not qualifying these 'affiliations' spatio-temporally nor specifying the psychological content of the resulting relationships. 'Affiliative', then, does not inform us of the degree of spatio-temporal or psychological closeness in any specific relationship which would help distinguish it from the 'distant' placement of the litigant subjects of legal rights and obligations. It is as if 'affiliation' were not the adjective of 'relationships' but the other way around. Two questions emerge at this point. First, Gilligan's abstract 'affiliative relationships' seem to signify emphatically, but also only 'abstractly', the idea of proximity as 'affiliation'. What does 'affiliation' mean when it is thought of in the abstract? It means, perhaps, that the verbs 'to approach' or 'to adopt' or 'to include, make member of' have been activated but have not yet crystallised into a new proximity. Is this model like Lévinas' 'proximity without commitment' and 'engagement-through disengagement'?

The second question worth asking is whether the emphasis on affiliation and closeness necessarily means that affiliation is antithetical to the confrontation of adversarial law. This question is important to ask because on it depends the understanding of the alterity between the strictures of justice and the charity of care, namely their inseparability and simultaneity. In this regard Whitbeck has made constructive criticism of Gilligan's ethics of care (Whitbeck 1996). The lesson from Gilligan seems to be that medical law fails to do justice to the ethics of care because of its 'antagonistic' approach to ethical issues arising in the doctor-patient relationship, whereby the question is always 'who owns' the decision. Instead, medical law can and must adopt a more appropriate attitude whereby the question asked will be *how* treatment decisions are and should be reached. In this connection, Whitbeck points out that already before Gilligan's work, in the 1970s the male writer John Ladd attempted a systematic philosophical investigation of the language of 'prospective' responsibility that ran in a similar vein. Although in Whitbeck's and Ladd's approaches responsibility for the close other is taken as the central ethical concept, as in Gilligan's ethics of care there is still place for the consideration of rights, and even of 'quantifiable benefits' (utilities). Also, more importantly, as their work on issues arising from medical technology indicates, they are committed, unlike Gilligan, to address the doctor-patient relationship as at once private and public.

III
Shared treatment decision making[10]

Certain analytical moral philosophers have now undertaken the role of providing us with a clearer 'account' of how exactly medical law must be re-focused from 'which of the doctor and patient *owns* the decision' to *how* such decisions are made. However, as I will promptly show, such attempts are destined to fail to express in a manner that is ethically unambiguous that the unique ethics of care *are* universalisable, and therefore compatible with general principles and rules of justice. Rather, they constitute an attempt to 'reconcile the two notions' dialectically. Thus, when the question is raised as to how a treatment decision must be reached, the reply is as follows. The patient and the doctor are both entitled to a decisive role in the therapeutic process, albeit each in his domain and in different proportions according to, in the case of the patient, his ability to 'override' the doctor in the 'subjective' evaluation of therapeutic facts, and in the case of the doctor, his ability to override the patient's 'subjective choices' when the patient's *biological being* is at stake. I show, further, that these models are variations on the generic theme of the doctor-patient relationship as 'special' and 'inherently inoffensive'. In the so-called model of SDM, analysed here, this happens specifically through a privileging of the communicative potential between doctor-and-patient with the emphasis on the in 'sharing' of the therapeutic labour.

---

[10]For a general and acute introduction to this doctrine see also Bloor and Horobin 1975. For a more radical approach see Rothman 1991.

In this connection Dan W. Brock states already in the first chapter of his book that his model of 'Shared treatment Decision Making' (hereafter SDM) is meant to compensate for the inadequacies of the legal obsession with questions of 'right to decide' in the division of therapeutic labour between doctor and patient (Brock 1993). His model involves a moral/philosophical account of this relationship whereby the so-called 'medical objectivism' (or 'paternalism') and 'patient subjectivism' views of treatment-decision-making are supposedly reconciled. It also calls for an end to medical law's obsession with the strict separation of therapeutic labour between self-determinant patient and medical professional in terms of the objectivist/subjectivist divide. The divide between objectivist/subjectivist treatment decision-making, Brock says correctly, belongs to the legacy of positivist theory which had wrongly insisted on a relatively sharp distinction between descriptive and empirical claims on the one hand, and evaluative claims and ethics on the other.[11] Thus, under 'medical objectivism' the diagnostic (descriptive) and therapeutic (empirical) statements of physicians in connection with the physical health of the patient are not comparable with the non-rational evaluation of the treatment by the patient, since the concepts of 'health' and 'disease' were mistakenly taken to be 'value-free' empirical or factual concepts. Thus conceived, the physician is thought to be an 'incorrigible' arbiter of the patient's health-related good.[12] Conversely, the patient-centred or 'subjectivist' model asserts the patient's 'incorrigibility' on the basis that physicians are not in a position to 'value' reliably what is in a patient's best interests in terms of subjective well-being (Buchanan 1991). Hence, it is believed that the patient ought to be the final arbiter of treatment, and his or her role should not be restricted to evaluating the physician's diagnosis and treatment-suggestions in the light of his or her own beliefs and moral convictions for the purpose of consenting to what is medically proposed. Rather these beliefs and values should form the objective of the treatment from the start, and bind the doctor's action.

In connection to the 'incorrigibility' argument, on the 'subjectivist' side of the doctor-patient opposition, Brock examines most modern philosophical accounts of the 'good life'. These seem to be in line with the subjectivist approach to patients' 'well-being', but when scrutinised in the context of care for suffering, they all fail.

---

[11]This distinction presupposes that moral or ethical judgements lack 'cognitive content', but are expressions of emotions or attitudes that are 'highly subjective' and can neither be true nor false, correct nor mistaken. Because no evaluative statements were held to be logically entailed by any descriptive or empirical scientific statements, moral reasoning was thought to be properly understood, not as reasoning, but as attempts at non-rational persuasion.

[12]Indeed Brock is correct in pointing out that the 'incorrigibility' thesis has often come to the defence of medical objectivism. A review of literature shows that even today many theorists continue to base their support for the objectivist model of treatment-decision-making on such views (Boorse 1975, 1977, 1987. Kass 1985).

They include all theories that focused on the problem of justification of moral judgement based on assumptions of 'meta-ethical subjectivity' as well as 'normative subjectivity'. With regard to the former, Brock looks at modern 'hedonist' theories[13] of the good for persons.[14] He is less than original in objecting that '[P]ersons are often mistaken about what will bring them pleasure or make them happy; others are often in a better position to determine this for them'.[15] With regard to the so-called 'meta-ethics' he examines 'preference satisfaction' theories of the good of persons, and correctly points out that these can only justify as being 'incorrigible' preferences for their own sake (therefore even misinformed preferences) and actual desires.[16] He points out how not even proponents of preference satisfaction theories would be prepared to defend a patient's desire for a particular treatment based on a false belief about his or her medical condition. Indeed, preference satisfaction theories become inconsequential. In the event of the clinical affair '[one] must allow for some correcting or 'laundering' of [the patient's] actual preferences' (Brock 1993: 66).[17] Finally, Brock looks at attempts to qualify juridically a patient's absolute right to decide. J. Rawls' 'reflective

---

[13]By terming these 'modern' hedonistic theories I wish to distinguish them from the Greek *Epicurean* doctrine. In the latter the emphasis is on avoiding suffering, not on pursuing pleasure. Thus to the extent that desire may be harmful it too must be avoided.

[14]What is common to hedonist theories is that they take the ultimate good for persons to be certain kinds of conscious experiences. The particular kinds of conscious experiences are variously characterised as pleasure, happiness, or the satisfaction or enjoyment that typically accompanies the successful pursuit of one's aims and desires.

[15]As Daniels (1988) has pointed out, incorrigibility is never achievable for moral judgements at a particular point in time. There is no assurance that new experiences, considerations or arguments may not in the future upset that equilibrium and cause some of the moral judgements it encompasses to be revised. Similarly Brock observes: 'Coherence accounts of justification in morality do make justified moral judgments ultimately subjective, in the sense that the moral judgments that are justified for a particular person are those that person makes in reflective equilibrium. Since reflective equilibrium is only an ideal at which a person can aim rather than a state one could be assured of being in before considering a significant ethical choice, *there is no reason to assume at the outset of shared decision making that the relevant values a patient brings to that decision making are maximally justified for him or her having survived reflective equilibrium*'. (Brock 1993: 63; my emphasis).

[16]Preference theories share a subjectivity with hedonist theories since they, too, make a person's good depend ultimately on what that particular person desires or prefers. They differ from hedonist theories in that they make the person's good depend on the realisation of the person's desired or preferred object alone, independently of any feelings of satisfaction or pleasure that may or may not accompany this realisation.

[17]'Nevertheless, the need for corrections of preferences makes clear that even the basic desires or preferences patients express in treatment decision making have no claim to incorrigibility in defining their good until they have either been corrected or it has been determined that they need no correction' (Brock 1993: 66).

equilibrium' thesis is one such meta-ethical coherentist theory which can be used to determine if a patient's view of his suffering and what is to be done about it is 'in line' with this patient's long-held view of the good (Rawls 1973, 1986). In this regard Brock, correctly, argues that:

> No plausible coherentist view gives any reason for physicians to accept as incorrigible patients' judgements about their good, or even the ultimate values by which patients define their good (Brock 1993: 63).

Let me come back to Brock's own premises. Although Brock says that absolute medical 'objectivity' is illusory, he also assumes that it is 'necessary' for patients to regard their doctors as if they could indeed be 'objective' in observing and analysing hard therapeutic 'facts'. The absolute right of the patient to decide their treatment, on the other hand, is far 'too abstract'; often the facts of an illness are too horrific to allow for judgement. As for the doctor's obligations, they are to be qualified in relation to the 'the role of the physician ... substantially defined by ethical commitments which are internal to medicine and to a significant degree, special to that profession ... since being a physician entails a commitment to a related and coherent body of ethical norms by which the profession in part judges itself and asks others to judge it' (Brock 1993: 71).[18] More specifically, Brock suggests that:

> *at least in principle* physicians can and should maintain the role of value-neutral facts provider, even if in practice they often fail to do so (ibid. 75; my emphasis).

This 'at least' is crucial in Brock's ideal model. It attaches itself to his belief that the aim of treatment-decision-making is that doctor and patient should 'share', and thus it spoils what could otherwise be a wonderful thesis. Such a thesis would have placed emphasis on the doctor-patient relation but *not* as traffic of information between 'subjectively suffering' patient and an 'objectively needed' doctor, who is thus 'needed' as a 'health mechanic' might be. It would go against Brock's view of the patient as an accumulation of physical and psychological needs and conscious interests which span what he calls an 'objective-subjective continuum'. And it would expose how Brock *simultaneously* presupposes that the exercise of patient self-determination ultimately depends on certain 'primary functional capacities', without which the patient's 'jurisdiction over his or her life' as it were lapses. For Brock the idea of the patient as unique subject is meaningful, and therefore the patient's opinion matters *only* if the patient enjoys a minimum level of 'biological and physical functioning' (ibid. 69). Brock's

---

[18] Thus a doctor's primary ethical duties are owed to his fellow medical professionals, his obligation to his patient merely being to apply his training and skills with competence and diligence to ensure attainment of the unshakable goal of full health.

formulation is, of course, circular, since the 'primariness' of the functional capacities he presumes are only 'primary' with regard to his essential 'different functionings that are a part of the good for persons' which fall at different points on the 'objective-subjective continuum' (Brock 1993: 76).

Therefore, there is a presupposition in the SDM model that when a patient lacks or has deficient 'primary functional capacities' he or she is to be seen as a subject in need of being treated as therapeutic object. Is this really something that the patient 'needs' or something that the carer does in an emergency? Let me offer an example. Already the ability of a doctor and a court to infer an 'implied consent'[19] to treatment of a patient in an emergency obscures the ways in which an 'emergency' affects the carer. The emphasis on a fictitious and legerdemain consent by the patient falsely imputes to the vulnerable patient a capacity to remain self-responsible in spite of the emergency. The doctor, in turn, is presented as if capable of restricting his or her tendency to intervene. As we saw, in order to bypass the doctor's subjective role courts go as far as demanding the discovery of the will of a comatose patient *even* where it is known that prior to the emergency the patient was legally incompetent.[20] In English law, as Kennedy and Grubb show, such logical atrocities are avoided because the judges deride the 'artificial' nature of implied consent and opt more often for the principle of necessity (Kennedy and Grubb 1994: 103). However, they continue, it is unclear whether the principle of 'necessity' is used like *estoppel* - as it ought to be. For instance, in cases of non-consented sterilisation of mentally ill women (see also earlier, at my Chapter 3) the principle of necessity is qualified by the test of the patient's 'best interests' in a way that makes it appear more than a case of implied consent. The correct question to ask is, *whose* necessity? given that the aim of applying for the sanctioning of enforced sterilisation is to end another person's ability to procreate, an important feature of the operation being that it is generally intended to be irreversible.[21]

Nevertheless, at the moment the SDM model appears to be the response of liberal ideology to the problem of 'useless' suffering; for example, it is this model which lies behind the recent reform in the law of incompetence, as discussed in Chapter 2. It represents the desire to communicate as the corner-stone of the doctor-patient relationship. As such, it flies in the face of most phenomenological accounts of sociality with the ill, which have insisted on the impossibility of establishing a 'common communicative environment' between doctor and patient (for literature on this issue see Chapter 3, n. 61). 'Communication' as flow of information presupposes intentionality, but the intentional perspectives from

---

[19]For the original modern decision on 'implied consent' see Mohr *v* .*Williams* (1905) 104 NW 12 (Sup Ct Minn.) as cited in Kennedy and Grubb 1994: 90-91.

[20]See Chapter 1, the *Saikewitcz* case.

[21]While modern micro-surgery makes it possible to reverse the operation in certain circumstances, this would defeat the primary purpose of sterilisation.

which a physician and a patient will respectively focus on the 'problem at hand' will differ greatly. A doctor and a patient cannot share the same intentional goals - even when a patient is a doctor. They inhabit 'different worlds'.[22]

This communication gap is, however, compatible with the idea of alterity between the doctor as unique carer and the patient as unique sufferer. Beyond communication there is involuntary expression and substitution. Alterity is cancelled when either the patient or the doctor is elevated to the status of incorrigible *ex-officio* judge of suffering or subject of self-redress, in which case either is then presented as indifferent to the absurdity of suffering. The SDM model, too, appears indifferent to such alterity. It is as if the parties have an 'obligation' to persuade each other to buy into their version of the meaning of suffering. When this fails, dispute remains inevitable. Brock explicitly states that in cases of patient-doctor disagreement the initiative could be with the doctor to ask the patient to 'sign him out' of responsibility 'AMA' - against medical advice (Brock 1993: 77). This, of course, is what already happens. SDM seems designed to explain why medical litigation is restricted to only a few cases. Moreover Brock's reformulating of the aim of treatment concedes that the therapeutic subject is first and foremost a therapeutic object. The idea is that once natural illness has reduced the patient to a passive object of suffering, the patient can only accede anew to the status of a subject through being objectified once more, this time 'therapeutically', by the physician. In so far as the doctor is concerned, Brock's model has no space for what I called 'counter-intentional' acts. Thus, if Lévinas is right that such acts constitute the pre-originary opening of subjectivity to the other, the physician's subjectivity seems banished from ethical proximity. Objectivism and subjectivism are opposed in binary fashion within the same discourse that establishes an ideal mastery of consciousness over suffering and responsibility for suffering. In other words, it is a discourse that reduces the significance of suffering to its phenomenal meaningfulness for the consciousness of either the doctor or the patient.

These models appeal to law because they idealise treatment decision making as if neutral towards the effects of 'useless' suffering or 'suffering for nothing'. Ideally, 'useless' suffering is conceived of as if always an opportunity for a neutral decision by the same self. This ideal has been expressed in modern terms as

---

[22]As K. S. Toombs has summarised the position: 'successful communication [between patient and practitioner] also presupposes a certain taken-for-granted congruence in the interpretational schemes of the communicators ... in the doctor-patient relationship this assumption is problematic ... [F]ull identity of the interpretational schemes is impossible in principle (since such schemes are determined by the unique biographical situation of the communicators). Any successful communication is, thus, dependant upon the communicators sharing a similar system of relevances ... [H]owever, doctor and patient do not share a substantially similar system of relevances with regard to the patient's illness' (Toombs 1992: 24-25).

defending patient autonomy.[23] Yet, as I have shown, the ideally self-determinate patient is only the offshoot of medico-scientific objectivism which in the modern era attempted to separate medical care from the act of offering relief with no therapeutic effect. Aristotle would deride the act of care for the other as lacking *endelecheia*, i.e. the status of self-aiming, and therefore, 'perfect activity', that is, living a 'good life' (Aristotle [1987: 28]). But it appears that in the modern era scientific medicine *did* finally accede, at least ideally, to the 'good life' of *endelecheia*, by denying and even suppressing its 'appetite for compassion'. A doctor acts only to cure; or, when that is impossible, he or she uses the terminal case as a source of knowledge. The modern patient, equally, resolves to decide what is best for him or herself 'in spite' of his or her multiple vulnerabilities (to illness, to medical manipulation). This is a Dante-esque vision of treatment-decision-making whereby, as in *Vita Nova*, the resolve to 'speak of' one's suffering and, moreover, the will to *decide* in spite of death and absurd suffering, allows the subject to become a poet, passing into a 'new life' where, nevertheless, he expects to remain self-same.

IV
False witness

Let me take a different perspective. I want to argue that the noted abeyance of the rule of law in the area of medical law and, in particular the policy of de-criminalising duality in judicial policy, must also be seen and explained *as a form of implication* in certain fundamental aspects of the judgement in the matter of crime. As I have already suggested, and this will be further substantiated in the discussion of the doctrine of informed consent in the next chapter, judges do their best to keep doctor-patient disputes out of court. In short, not only is criminal conviction unlikely but courts are reluctant to adjudicate complaints by patients in civil suits. In fact, I argue, the two attitudes are linked. The undermining of the medical civil suit occurs through an implicit 'criminalisation' of the civil suit proceedings. This, I submit, takes the form of restricting the 'contest of meanings' amongst plural interpretations of the concepts related to illness-suffering (hurt, pain, risk etc.).

---

[23] Thus I. Berlin states: 'I wish my life to depend on myself, not on external forces of whatever kind. *I wish to be the instrument of my own*, not of other men's acts of will. I wish to be a subject not an object; to be moved by reasons, by conscious purposes which are my own, not by causes which affect me, as it were, from outside. I wish to be somebody, not anybody; a doer - deciding not being decided for, self-directed and not acted upon *by external nature or by other men* ... I wish, above all, to be conscious of myself as a thinking, willing, active being, bearing responsibility for his choices and able to explain them by reference to his own ideas and purposes' (Berlin 1969: 123).

The confrontation of doctor and patient in court is also discouraged. Thus, a true legal dialogue over the limitations of the premises and principles of medical law is eliminated, as judges, especially under the influence of SDM principles, act in favour of unilaterally 'incorrigible' treatment-decision-makers on the matter of the meaning of illness-suffering (e.g. the *Bolam* test in English law whereby the standards of medical care are left to be defined by doctors, just as with any other profession). Moreover, as I show in more detail later in the analysis of *Sidaway*, it is just as possible that judges will react to SDM principles by amplifying patients rights as it is that they will deny them. At first, this restrictive attitude of 'law' seems odd, given that the 'law' is particularly good at opposing 'paternalist medicine' to 'subjectivist patients', 'siding' alternately with the one or the other. On a different level, one may speak metaphorically of a legal 'allergy' to the peculiar 'object' of human suffering. It is my argument that this 'suffering' is avoided because it does *more* than just offer itself to an argument from 'multiple points of view', ranging from the scientific account of 'hard' facts to the patient's subjectively incorrigible account of their 'well-being' and their individual needs. The failure of medical law to encourage, and in reverse, the activity of suppressing, the 'legally useless' and 'uninteresting' moral confrontation between patient and doctor indicates a certain legal aversion to the very subject of non-objectifiable 'suffering' and responsibility.

Following Lévinas' phenomenology of suffering I have said that the patient is not merely the 'owner of', but also a 'witness' to his or her suffering. However, *so* is the 'external' observer, e.g. the doctor. This irreducible tension would be denied if either one is assumed to be an 'expert' witness, or an 'incorrigible' judge of suffering, either from a thoroughly 'subjective' point of view or from an objective one. In the case of English law, which embraces 'medical paternalism', the absolute decision-maker is the scientific doctor, as if an *ex-officio* incorrigible judge of suffering.[24] The scientific doctor, moreover, is thus conceived as relating directly to the 'object' of suffering, as if exclusively authorised to apprehend it as 'disease'. The patient of such a doctor, in turn, is thought of as no more than witness to the 'public crime' of illness, reporting on its suffering with much less authority than its symptoms present directly to the trained eye; and almost as passive an object for medico-scientific decisionism as a broken machine is for a mechanic. On the other hand, in North America, whilst the patient is said to be the decisive decision maker *qua* consumer, courts seem prepared, as I have noted earlier, to side-line patient's consent and rights if their exercise would be 'unreasonable', and/or if the doctor makes use of the 'therapeutic privilege' available to him whereby the patient can be lied to if the doctor predicts that the patient will over-react to 'bad news', so that he may become less co-operative in his treatment.

---

[24]For an example of how the notion of 'medical paternalism' is used, see Childless 1983.

A comparison comes to mind: perhaps we could say that in some instances the doctor acts like a criminal prosecutor who, upon hearing of the news of an injury from a victim who claims the right to self-defence, is capable of initiating proceedings independently of the victim's will. In declaring his wishes to his doctor the patient is not in relation to the latter. In being simultaneously the 'victim' of illness and the judge of his/her 'own suffering' the self-determinate patient is, literally, expected to be ready for intense 'self-redress'. However, neither in England nor in North America are judges happy to see their courts turned into an arena where the intrinsic absurdity of human suffering can be debated, and where the paradoxical nature of responsibility for absurd suffering can be evoked. For this reason, medical suits lose their character of civil dispute, as either doctor or patient is implicitly elevated to the status of 'incorrigible judge' of the non-sense that is suffering and responsibility for it. Affectivity beyond intentionality is thus obscured. The 'assimilation' of the non-sense of suffering in the subjectivist patient judgement, but also in the 'objectivist medical judgement', correspond to a 'sovereign' subject of consciousness acting with the 'authority' associated with being's persistence in Being, in self-identity and self-coincidence, without interruption or surprise. In all this, medical law has become the 'false witness' of human suffering and responsibility, and therefore, their proximity.

We have witnessed law's 'oscillation' with regard to proximity based on suffering in at least two forms: ambivalence as to the nature of the doctor-patient relationship and an implication in *and* disengagement of medical responsibility from criminal law. On one level this 'oscillation' of medical law towards the mystery of care shows a surprising, albeit involuntary, 'reciprocity' towards the mystery of proximity based on un-objectifiable and absurd human suffering. In Latin *reciprocus* indicates an arrested or self-cancelling movement at once back and forth (*re-co* + *pro-co*). Now, the earlier Greek root of Latin *procum* also suggests the 'sudden immediacy of surprise' (Papanikolaou 1989: 343). However, this surprise is cancelled in so far as medical law refuses to conceive of the subjectivity of counter-intentionality as the basis of its own legal subject of rights and obligations. This renders difficult the proper adjudication of patient complaints. In response, judges attempt to overcome the problem of non-sensical human suffering and responsibility by giving a 'criminal edge' to the medical civil suit. One of the parties is proclaimed an incorrigible, self-contained judge of suffering, at the cost of de-subjectivising the other party, and is expected to endow suffering with a definitive meaning. What, in conclusion, must we retain from the simultaneous 'criminalisation' of the doctor-patient dispute *and* the more real decriminalisation of its outcome? The two coincide in that, in both cases, the 'useless' or un-measurable human suffering is not responded to in disinterested 'engagement through disengagement', but is 'made use of' for the purpose of making sense of the doctor's or the patient's self as closure or consciousness, being-for-itself capable of new vitality and inexhaustible virility even in the event of witnessing the non-sense which oppresses it.

V

In the matter of 'informed consent': how the object of medico-legal interest is the patient's soul-less *being*

As noted earlier, in theory medical intervention to which the patient has not offered a free and fully informed consent renders the doctor liable in Tort and Criminal Law.[25] Any problems with the doctrine must be seen as part of the wider judicial difficulty in conceptualising the overall function of consent in the doctor-patient relationship, which as I have shown remains ambiguous (contractual/fiduciary). To reproduce the sense of uncertainty let me briefly recount an episode. In the space of a few months, the same judge in two different cases presented patient consent as both a granted licence and as a defensive armament. Thus in *Re R,* involving a minor whose parents had first given their consent for its treatment but later withdrew it, Lord Donaldson, intent on allowing the treatment to proceed, said that consent is like 'a key which unlocks a door' which 'can be used repeatedly and cannot be withdrawn' (as cited in Kennedy and Grubb 1994: 105).[26] Later, in *Re W,* he said that:

> [Consent] has two purposes, the one clinical and the other legal ... On reflection I regret my use in *Re R* of the key-holder analogy ... because keys can lock as well as unlock. ... I now prefer the analogy of the legal 'flak jacket' which protects [doctors] from claims by the litigious [patients].[27]

The judicial policy to create exceptions to legal norms especially for the doctor-patient relationship is particularly evident in the courts' attempt to restrict the scope of the doctrine of 'informed consent' which requires a doctor to give the patient a detailed and intelligible diagnosis and state all risks and alternatives. It is interesting that the demand for a wider interpretation of this doctrine has initially come from non-lawyers, especially from medical sociologists and moral philosophers, and was only later echoed in jurisprudence (G. Dworkin 1982, R. Dworkin 1993) and 'black-letter' medical law commentary (Kennedy and Grubb 1994; my Chapter 3). This already indicates a certain legal indifference towards the subject of 'consent' although it is also thought of as the very 'backbone' of liberal medico-legal doctrine. This indifference is most indicative of the ethical attitude of lawyers towards the issue of the ethical freedom of subjectivity to intervene, by means of 'good violence', for the suffering other, as well as its concomitant obligation to assume responsibility for its compassionate 'violence'. I do not believe that responsibility in these cases can be seen merely as a problem of

---

[25] For an exposition of the general legal premises see G. Dworkin 1982.

[26] *Re R (a minor) (wardship: consent to treatment)* [1992] Fam 11; as cited in Kennedy and Grubb 1994: 105.

[27] *Re W (a minor) (medical treatment)* [1992] 4 All E.R. 627; ibid.

information-exchange and communication between patient and scientific doctor. For me, medical responsibility emerges primarily as ethical duty to commit compassionate 'violence'. Let me therefore make it clear that I am not interested in arguing either for a wider or a for narrower scope of informed consent. Instead, I am interested in how the various interpretations of the doctrine are the judiciary's way of imposing limits on responsibility for the infinite, non-sense of vulnerability of being.

The notion of patients' 'informed consent' has been de-limited, in recent interpretations, in ways which obscure the magnitude and scope of physicians responsibility for their interventions - independently of the 'amount of information' that they have disclosed and shared with the patient about his/her condition or treatment. The most important aspect of the problem of 'patient' consent is that - more than any other kind of consent - it shows the 'nakedness' of the legal subject whose 'consent' is as much a sign of freedom as of subjugation. As we have seen, medical law's concept of the 'autonomous patient' rather obscures this nakedness and the surprising reactions it occasions. We have seen examples of this in the case of PVS patients (Chapter 1), and patients with hysterical delusions and the determination to persist in them (Chapter 2). More than anything, such patients are never *in extremis* but always assumed to speak for themselves *through* their 'meaningful' suffering - which is to say they are expected to swallow their agony and talk.

It is my argument that effectively, English medical law on consent has been interpreted in the leading case, analysed below, in ways which penalise the patient who fails to ask persistently for detailed information from his/her doctor, whilst excusing the doctor who fails to volunteer disclosure. The relevant English law was laid down in *Sidaway*.[28] There, no means were too strenuous in order to dismiss Ms Sidaway's claim that her *total paralysis*, following an operation, was attributable to her doctor's negligence, since he had been aware of the risk of paralysis but had failed to disclose it, and so had arguably disabled her from making an informed choice.[29] Ms Sidaway's predicament of utter passivity and paralysis of bodily expressivity is just as grave as that of a comatose patient, although it is *reversed*. Yet, the court in *Sidaway* accepted the medical opinion that the patient's paralysis had only realised a risk 'too small' to deserve prior disclosure by the doctor. According to Kennedy and Grubb *Sidaway* pays only lip service to the certainty of the law. The two commentators are puzzled that, on the

---

[28]*Sidaway v. Board of Governors of the Bethlem Royal Hospital* [1985] AC 871, [1985] 1 All E.R. 643; ibid.
[29]Causation, the use of expert evidence as to accepted medical practice, and a renewed emphasis on the 'best interests' principle were all used. Further, the final decision to dismiss the appeal due to 'insufficient evidence' has a sinister undertone since at the time of the trial the doctor in question had passed away and the patient was the only viable source of evidence.

one hand, the decision seems to restate authoritatively the *Bolam* principle whereby the standard of care is a matter of medical judgement; whilst on the other hand, only one of the judges was unequivocal on this point. Of the others, Lord Templeman kept a safe distance,[30] whilst Lord Bridge said that the 'issue whether non-disclosure ... should be condemned as a breach of the doctor's duty of care is an issue to be decided *primarily* on the basis of expert medical evidence, applying the *Bolam* test'. Similarly at the Court of Appeal Sir John Donaldson MR had said that the proper standard is that 'which is *rightly* accepted as proper by a body of skilled and experienced medical men'. Since the *Bolam* principle is said to be 'unequivocal', what we must understand by 'primarily' is anybody's guess.

In this regard, attention must be paid to the clarificatory statement (I use the word euphemistically) by the court that it could 'potentially' move beyond the *Bolam* and 'override the standards set by established medical practice' in the event that a doctor 'blunders' in failing to disclose a 'grave risk'. Now the gravity of risk can be measured either in probabilistic terms, in which case it is strictly a scientific problem, or, in terms of its 'subjective' *impact* on the patient. The latter too is usually determinable either objectively (in terms of medically defined 'health') or subjectively (in terms of well-being). In declaring their determination to overrule scientific assessment of the seriousness of the possible impact and side-effects of the treatment on the patient's health in case of 'blunder', the judges could not be talking of statistics. Their main concern was to create a framework in which the contrasting (objective-subjective) views of seriousness can be reconciled in the view of law's 'reasonable man'. Therefore, since Ms Sidaway's total paralysis was not found by the judges to be so 'reasonably grave' to deserve disclosure, one must assume that only threats to the patient's physical *existence* would be allowed. Moreover, perhaps not *even* if the risk had been 'permanent vegetative state' would the court have been motivated to proclaim that the doctor's non-disclosure was, in principle, unlawful according to *law's* reason. In conclusion, the judges will effectively challenge the reasonableness of good medical practice *only* in so far as it may destroy the patient as a 'living thing', i.e. as the therapeutic *object* around which modern medicine revolves as the closed system of curative science, but not short of that point.

In other words, it appears that judicial interest is confined to risks to the patient's *biological life* whilst indifference is shown to her subjectivity. Since Ms Sidaway had survived the operation, and so had remained a 'therapeutic object' - in fact even more of an 'object' following the operation which resulted in her total paralysis - the standards of care are left to medicine and her appreciation of the changes in the quality of her life leave the judges unimpressed. The situation will

---

[30]In this connection Kennedy and Grubb emphasise the disjunction in the judge's reasoning, that 'I do not subscribe to the theory that the patient is entitled to know everything [about her treatment] *nor* to the theory that the doctor is entitled to decide everything' (Kennedy and Grubb 1994: 185).

only marginally differ in the case of risky psychological treatments.[31] One conclusion is that whilst the law refuses to punish doctors for not volunteering information disclosure above the professional standards, it nevertheless obliges them to answer truthfully any number of questions asked by the patient. In effect, the law thus penalises the patient for not taking the initiative in asking questions concerning treatment-related risks. This situation is similar to the legal treatment of the victim of criminal rape when she is alleged to have failed to have made explicit to the perpetrator her refusal to intercourse. Hence there is no legal protection for patients who in remaining idle or silent 'provoked' their doctor to keep them uninformed and treat them as if they were broken machines.

What is law's function with regard to being's 'disinterested engagement with its other as otherwise than being/not being'? It is not just that law cannot express this ethical relation in its principles and doctrines. Medical law, in particular, is the symptom of a legal system which not only fails to *express* all the ethical or less-ethical violence which is involved in the being-for-each-other, but also *proscribes* the exposure of subjectivity to absurd suffering and the responsibility this demands. Rather, an attitude of relative moral indifference, often verging on utter 'blindness', is *actively imposed*. As I showed in the case above, but also in all the others I have examined earlier, this is first achieved through the use of norms which except from their application that which is seen as 'excessive' suffering or vulnerability of the human being, and, simultaneously, ban or foreclose the subject of pure emotion, obsessive compassion and counter-intentionality from the realm of its responsibility - which is ethically perverse because 'justice is inseparable from charity' and, in consequence, liability for intentional or negligent harm is merely an instance of gratuitously extended responsibility for all that the other suffers even if as a result of their own fault or 'naturally'.

---

[31]Arguably, the implication of *Sidaway* for 'psychological' treatments is that courts may be prepared to overrule established opinion and accept that the psychologist 'blundered' by not disclosing risks, but only in cases where the psychological impairment of the patient amounts to disenabling the patient psychologically to be subjected to further treatment.

CHAPTER 5

The 'Naked Being':
A Face (Non-persona) Grata

Someone's son has died. Respond: that is beyond our power, so it is not an evil. Someone's father has disinherited him. What do you think about it? It is beyond our power, it is not an evil. He was distressed about it. That does concern us, it is an evil. He bore it courageously. That concerns us, it is good (Epictetus, cited by M. Foucault in Rabinow 1994: 104).

The original rapport between law and life is not the application [of norms to facts], but *Abandonment* [of facts by norms] (Agamben 1997: 37).

[In order to] envisage [absurd] suffering from an inter-human perspective ... [whereby suffering] is meaningful within me [but] is useless for my other [*sensée en moi, inutile en autrui*] ... [one must abandon] a point of view of relativity in relation to suffering ... [However] The inter-human perspective ... may be lost in the order of politics of the City where the Law establishes the mutual obligations of the citizens. ... The order of politics - post-ethical or pre-ethical - which inaugurates the 'social contract' is neither the insufficient condition nor the necessary end of ethics. In its ethical position, the me is distinct from the citizen ... [but also from] the individual who precedes all order in pure, natural egoism ... (EN: 118; my translation).

I
The constitutive ethical perversity of modern law

Let us assume that by the term 'society' we indicate both 'horizontally'-structured reciprocal social relationships, comprising multiple subjects of law, and the 'vertical' relationships of being-for-my-other, whereby one subject exercises, *anarchically* and *disinterestedly*, power, mastery and control over another, e.g. parenthood, love, teaching, giving succour and caring. It is my argument that 'justice' and 'ethical proximity' occupy the intersection of the two kinds of relationship. The legal 'judgment' (which I have spelled without a second 'e' to distinguish the law's supposed 'impersonality' and neutrality and timelessness), represents solely the horizontal order, and it is memory and the re-enactment of its principles, rules and measures. On a sociological level 'society' is a system in which, despite temporary turbulences, the distant remains distant and the close remains close; there is exchange, transformation and revolution, but not mixing of difference; ontological time takes over and it keeps as still as dust that has settled. On the other hand, the personalised event of 'judgement' signifies an assumption of responsibility which can only be explained as of the 'vertical' and 'one-way' kind of association between self and other. In the end, there is only judg(e)ment. In this connection the notion that 'ethical proximity is inseparable from justice' helps to illuminate how 'being-with-others', in or outside law, is interrupted by the anarchy of being-*for-my*-other, which unsettles the ontological dust and displaces the binary opposition between an abstractly established social order and the concrete responsibility of specifically situated subjects of history.

Arguably, legal judgment becomes possible at the 'intersection' of the vertical and horizontal levels of action and decision. The legal judgment, that is, does not appear as synthesis between the two perspectives mentioned above, and therefore can be neither only 'objective' judgment nor merely 'subjective' judgement. Rather the juridical decision as judg(e)ment represents subjectivity's ability to produce an intersection between universality and individuation. There is emission and gratuitous expenditure of judg(e)ment by the *me* of each one of us which comes to exist outside essence, *for* a unique other. This points to a 'society' consisting of individual lovers, parents and neighbours who, respectively, fall in love, become impregnated with responsibility, and synchronise their egos, not 'in order to avert war' but for *humanity*'s sake. To be sure, the giver of personalised judgement 'violently acts on' the other being, with the force of a subject of consciousness which is full of 'content', a history and a culture; moreover, he/she does so with an urgency that exceeds his/her own memory and power of projection. Thanks to the desire for uniqueness and *disinterestedness*, he or she is bound to abstract the 'other' it encounters at the intersection, and to 'extract' him or her with 'ethical violence' from placement on the 'horizontal' order, suggesting him or her to be 'higher'. Regarding this elevation, although my 'non-intentional charity' and 'compassion' cannot 'absolve' an other from his or her responsibilities to third parties by means of the aforementioned abstraction, it is my argument that (as I illustrate in section II below) without an obsessive act of charity there is *inadmissibility* of my other as 'unique' subject in the realm of justice which involves comparison and measure.

First, however, let me revisit my earlier observations in the light of the above. In my review of medical law I found that, in addition to proscribing affectivity-beyond-representation, law effectively imposes indifference towards the otherwise-than-being/non-being, since its descriptions are also prescriptive. The individual being is described alternatively, either as being-for-itself, essence and persistence in being with calculable and tradeable interests, or else as non-being, and death as nothingness, given entirely to the survivor's memory rather than to emotion. There is in this a certain denial of the human vocation of 'insatiable compassion', but also, the *anachronistic* act of presupposing a social 'order' as separate from, and prior to the anarchy of 'one-way' obsessions directed at abstractly 'unique' others. 'Disinterestedness' and 'engagement through disengagement' become, thus, inconceivable. In this connection, it must be said that there is a perversity in modern legal practice. Even if today's legal judg(e)ment, in the sense I gave earlier, turns against its own condition, that is, denies the violence of ethical proximity with the abstractly unique, 'non-object' of the judged person's Face, it cannot be reduced either to a merely subjective judgement or to an merely objective judgment, since each of these two 'depends' upon the other. I propose that what happens, rather, is that when the 'ethical violence' of a necessarily magisterial legal decision is not acknowledged, i.e. when personal responsibility lapses and 'authorities' for our one-way obsessions are searched for, erroneously, within the 'order' of society, there may occur a dangerous perversity - namely, that in our judg(e)ments in the above sense, for disinterestedness towards the unique other is substituted interest, or alternatively, indifference. Further, it is my argument that when this happens, i.e. when I imply that the other concerns *me* out of interest only, my own ethical subjectivity as well as my other's becomes an object of pure moral indifference.

The fact that law's description of what subjectivity is/is not operates prescriptively presents us with the problem of authority. However, as I have explained, the legal subject is not allowed to replace 'authorisation' for its actions or omissions upon another with the anarchy and radical affectivity of the being-for-the-other; as result, authority is sought in the false 'truths' about what 'is' and what 'is not'. Let me elaborate further on this kind of 'ontological' politics. Giorgio Agamben has recently presented us with a convincing view of a distinctively modern ontological system in which, essentially, what I have called absurd suffering and responsibility are 'excepted'. But let me explain. In his terms the 'juridico-political order' exists by excepting from social and normative interest the biological human life (Agamben 1995). In the *polis*, the 'nakedness' of individual 'raw life', as exposure to needs, sufferings and risks, must lose its significance and becomes 'suspended', subject to *selective* normative focus, or in my terms, to 'interest' alternating with the indifference of 'turning a blind eye'. I submit that Agamben's 'excepted' raw life refers to what, for Lévinas and for myself, would be the 'non-object' of the disinterested, or counter-intentionally charitable self, i.e. to the idea of being as other than what is engaged with out of interest, or ignored in pure indifference.

Agamben draws his argument from Aristotle's *Politics,* and focuses on the crucial distinction that the Greeks of Aristotle's time drew between *zoe,* the basic fact of living which is common to animals and humans and gods, and *bios*, the form or way of living of a particular human individual in a group (Agamben 1995: 10). Let me paraphrase slightly what Agamben says in order to make apparent how close his thesis is to mine, although, of course, our conclusions are different. Agamben infers from the aforementioned strict Aristotelian distinction between 'life' and 'social being' that politics in the *polis* of the classical world was founded on the suspension of political interest from (or an imposition of indifference towards) the individual's survival and death. That is, political beings (and only they can be held 'responsible') supposedly must be blind to the vital (*zoe*-related) activity of being which persists in being-for-itself blindly (*le vivant*: the human as persistence in essence which is threatened by annihilation in death or, in yet different terms, the subject of symmetrical 'life and death instincts', *zoe* and *thanatos*). Zoe and its correlative notion of privacy rested entirely in the private domain of the *oikos*.

However (and in this connection Agamben reiterates Michel Foucault's thesis) in modernity 'naked life' becomes increasingly *politicised*.[1] For Agamben, this 'politicisation' of 'naked life' in modern western politics is not to be studied as merely the result of a historical 'transformation' in the last few centuries. Agamben asserts, and in this he extends Foucault's thesis on modernity, that the so-called 'bio-politics' were in place even before the advent of the Enlightenment. All in all, whilst Foucault's thesis explains the modern blurring of the classical distinction between private *zoe* and public *bios,* Agamben's focuses on the constitutive classical positing of these two terms in a relation of *ex-ceptio* or 'inclusive exclusion'. More specifically, being's unsocialised 'vitality' or 'animality', which as we saw correlates to Lévinas' *esse*, or being's persistence in Being, or being-for-itself), was always of 'interest' to political society. Agamben rightly asserts that the classical Aristotelian definition of *polis,* based as it is on the opposition between crude biological existence and living well with other humans (*zen* and *eu zen*), already constituted a relation of, so to speak, 'negative interest', which Agamben calls 'suspension' (Agamben 1995: 36); in short, to exclude from the realm of politics and responsibility that which is of no interest to collective well-being is also to 'include' it, albeit only in the form of an object of active indifference, i.e. that which *must* be excluded. In classical times, therefore, the 'solitary' fact of survival, persistence in being or *bios* of each singular existent is already included in the constitution of politics and responsibility, albeit in the form of 'exclusory inclusion' (ibid. 15). For Agamben, moreover, Aristotle's *Politics* offers evidence of the fact that western politics are constituted from the

---

[1]In analysing political power Foucault's thesis had abandoned the traditional juridico-institutional models (the definition of sovereignty, the theories of the state) for the sake of analysing concrete modalities through which power penetrates the subjects' bodies and forms of life. That is, the body and mind of the individual become the focus of totalising objective techniques (such as the science of policing) and the place of the deployment of individuating subjective strategies (such as 'technologies' of self-care regimes which are internalised by the individual in the process of subjectification). In short, 'modernity' is characterised by the 'transformation' (I use this term provisionally) of politics into 'bio-politics' where the individual as simple, living body exposed to constant 'natural' (and in my terms absurd) threats becomes the location for the 'exercise of state power' in post-modern conditions which are characterised by social and cultural 'fragmentation' and loss of the law-sovereignty model of governance; 'state power' is now 'governmental power' interested in the minutest risks to the health and well-being of individual beings whose happiness adds to the well-being of the social totality.

beginning by this 'exclusion (which is also an implication) of naked life' (ibid. 15). All in all:

> [T]he [individual's] naked life has, in western politics, the singular privilege of being that of which the exclusion founds the city (ibid.).

In my terms, Agamben's observation goes to show that already in 'Athens' the meaning of responsibility, in the political and legal sense, excludes disinterested engagement. But beyond this obvious point there lies a more interesting one. Agamben is right that 'the inclusion of *zoe* in the *polis* [is] in itself very ancient'; and I agree further that Foucault's 'modernity' is *not* characterised simply by the fact that life as such becomes an important object of calculations and provisions of state power (ibid. 17). To be sure, the specificity of late modernity consists rather in that, in it:

> naked life, originally situated in the margins of political organisation [as pure exception], progressively coincides with political life ... exclusion and inclusion, exterior and interior, *bios* and *zoe,* law and fact, enter into a zone of irreducible indifferentiation (ibid.).

In other words, in the 'gradual' process of consolidation of western political and juridical institutions - since classical Greece, but more importantly for law, since Roman times, there has also occurred an increase in political and normative interest in the individual's 'naked life'. From implicating it 'through exclusion', it seems the city now 'progressively' implicates it in socially meaningful life. The classical exception-alisation of being's 'nakedness' from politics and normativity constitutes an unethical conversion of disinterestedness into indifference. In modernity another 'option' is added for destroying disinterestedness: the taking of 'interest' in individual lives.

II
The *redundant* expulsion of ethical subjectivity

No stranger has had to spend the night in the street, for I have kept open a house for the traveller (Job 31:32).

[In Lévinas] Ethical obligation arises not from the logical and ontological universality of reason which discloses to knowledge criteria for freely determined action, but rather immediately from the uniqueness of the moral situation itself. In reversal of the classical order of privilege which promoted speculative reason, obligation is no longer first disclosed in its universality and intelligibility [as law, duty], known and then evaluated. On the contrary, moral obligation binds us because it takes hold *immediately*, before understanding or decision on the part of the subject. Such an absolute obligation properly defines the status of *prophetic* discourse which grounds itself solely on the authority of its source and bypasses the mediatory role of reason ... How is it possible to express in philosophical language a situation so strange that it takes place in the most extreme particularity, yet concerns the universal meaning of subjectivity? How is it possible to translate into 'Greek', that is, into philosophical language, this inspiration and this situation that belongs to prophetic eschatology? (Fabio Ciaramelli in Bernasconi *et al.*, eds. 1991: 85-86; my emphasis).

How is it possible to translate into 'Greek', that is, into philosophical language, this inspiration and this situation that belong to prophetic eschatology? I intend here to tackle the relevant difficulty. Instead of speculating how prophecy reverts to reason I wish to reverse the problem: how does reason revert to prophecy? To help me I will use a Greek myth, and ask how its reason reverts to prophecy; and how, despite its ontological language, it nevertheless speaks of the relation between subjectivity's moral obligation for charity and its duty to obey the law. Simultaneously, I will also point out once again how, as Lévinas says, justice and charity 'may appear strangers [to each other] if presented as successive stages [although] in reality they are inseparable and simultaneous'.

In particular I am attempting to trace the 'origins' of subjectivity and of law in an ancient Greek myth on the genesis of the criminal trial as it was incorporated in the last part of Aeschylus' trilogy *Agamemnon, The Libation-Bearers* and *Eumenides.*[2] Mythological drama is chosen over anthropology since I disagree with the premise that the modern subject can indeed discover its pre-legal constitution by means of recovering its (primitive) past. It is impossible to establish unmediated access to that 'past' and impossible to discover a tribal present. 'Discoveries' of this sort are more inventions that realise the intentions of the discoverer than re-constitutions of a lost 'natural' state of humankind.[3] Moreover, I, like any other subject of law, am constituted *in* law and therefore can

---

[2] I am using the translation by H. Weir Smyth and H. Lloyd-Jones 1926, 1930, 1956, 1952, 1957, 1963, 1983.

[3] In this light an explicitly mythical account of the origins of justice or law is more 'responsible' than a supposedly 'objective' anthropology which scans cultures and eras looking for structures. Yet I am not sure that honesty equals responsibility, as I have already said in Chapter 3 where I criticised Boyd-White's view that sincerity in a legal judgment is by itself ethical. Here, although Aeschylus speaks to his audience with poetic licence he is not entirely responsible in the above sense. His play pretends to seek the origin of formal Athenian justice in a by-gone, primitive era where a higher kind of proximity was still anticipating its encounter with legality. In his 'explanation' of how a jury trial became possible for the 'vile' crime of matricide Aeschylus not only incorporates a variety of myths describing ancient events (and for that matter in territories foreign to Athens), but moreover he elevates the 'facts' invoked in the myths to the higher status of absolute cause. From this, I believe, we may infer that the responsibility of 'honesty' decreases as honesty is assumed by intentionality.

only retroactively and anachronistically recall the 'original' moment of subjectivity's 'extra-legal', inaugural constitution. As the philosopher put it:

> all progressivist and evolutionary anthropology is false. The beginning is the strangest and the mightiest. What comes after that is not a development but flattening that results from me spreading out ... Historical knowledge is an understanding of the mysterious character of this beginning. If anything it is knowledge of mythology (Heidegger 1961: 155).

The myth in the *Eumenides* concerns the setting up of the 'first' criminal trial in ancient Athens for the sake of a stranger, Orestes, who having committed matricide, has been exiled from his native Argos.[4] Matricide was a crime so heinous that under Argos' customary law, there was no trial for it. In fact, it was not at all a penal 'crime' because the murder of the mother was still considered to be a superior abomination committed against the divine order. To this *hubris* corresponded the 'fate' of expulsion of the accused from his, as well any other city, with the certainty that cast away from proximity in exile the perpetrator would perish in utter deprivation, haunted by the 'madness-bearing' monstrous Furies. Thus, there was no need for legal sanction. *Hubris* and corresponding fate were two phenomena with an irreducibly marginal relation to the city's legal system. The *polis* of Argos, which had expelled its citizen Orestes, and Athens, which eventually received him - and in the process 'inaugurated' its criminal justice system - and their respective legal systems, appear, in this story, to have established and maintained a peculiar relationship with Orestes-in-exile.

In Argos, Orestes had been stripped of his right to a politically and legally meaningful self-identity. There remained of Orestes a being who continued to be 'interesting' to the *polis* of Argos, albeit as a simple living entity - after all his life had been spared; he had been abandoned, 'naked', utterly exposed to all kinds of risks, and was de-personified in the juridical sense. He had no access to the 'neutral standpoint of the law' from which he could retrieve his own past in law's

---

[4] I am focusing on the way myth is explored in a classical tragedy because I am intrigued by Walter Benjamin's distinction between tragedy and the modern 'mourning play' (*Trauerspiel*). In the first, the dramaturg is relatively free to assume an idea of time which is conclusively shaped by the form of the drama itself (a style which is very much evident in current so-called post-modern dramatic art). In it the individual hero holds a central place, for although 'fated', his or her fate is encapsulated at every point by the dramatic language. The moment counts singularly and cannot be deferred. By contrast in the mourning play (typified by Shakespearean theatre) the author presents an experience of unresolved time. The individual's fate remains inconclusive and is expressible only by means of allegory. Yet, in what follows it will become apparent that in a sense tragedy is already a mourning play. In any case, the aim of my serious play with the myth is not to decipher its significance in an Ancient Greek context, but to enquire the extent to which this dramatically explored myth 'is already enlightenment' (see, generally, the commentary of Jarvis 1998: 20-43).

memory, and assume his inherited place in the inter-*esse* of the *polis*. In short, for Argosians Orestes-in-exile was no longer an 'individual' in the sense that, although he was 'there', he was no longer a *member* of the social totality. Thus, with the penumbra of totality gone, his being could make no claim to individuality: he was 'different' but not singular; such being is thought of as still maintaining its essence, in the simple sense of persisting in being, but only as object of moral indifference by others. Anyone could kill Orestes without punishment. Indeed, Orestes attaches to no particular identity. The wandering Orestes of Aeschylus' drama is in fact nameless and anonymous. For the Argos legal system Orestes is a 'no-body' who, nevertheless, 'makes all the difference'. Subjectivity in exile is condemned to bear the distinguishing feature of the *rejected* in perpetuity. In exile, subjectivity cannot turn to anyone for help. He or she will be treated as someone who did not so much 'lose his place' in the home-town through accident or fault, but who *embodies rejection*. Orestes is therefore also the 'polluted' subject from whose absurd fate all sane others must keep clear. Criminals sent into perpetual exile constituted an exception not only from the norms of the city in which they committed the crime, but also from the pan-Hellenic divine law of hospitality (*philoxenia* or the love of strangers). Because Orestes was so 'polluted' all proximity with him was dangerous; so much so that no-one could have 'cleansed' him from his pollution by means of ritual sacrifice (it took the god Apollo's 'coup' to perform such a purification in Delphi, and even that was later contested in court as invalid purification by the Erinyes).

In this connection, it is interesting that Giorgio Agamben also focuses on the Roman law institution of *Homo Sacer,* i.e. the human who can be killed with impunity, albeit not in a ritual fashion. What is unique about this institution is that it represents a view of life as *both* excluded and included in the interests of the *polis*. More precisely, in this institution Roman law endorses 'raw life' in the juridico-political order positively but does so exclusively in the form of exception to normativity: law authorises anyone to kill an individual branded *Homo Sacer* without any legal penalty, for whatever reason and in any manner (except in religious sacrifice). For the first time, and only as that which the *polis* excludes, *zoe* becomes an object of legally sanctioned murder, but with no political significance and 'outside' the realm of responsibility. The biological life of *Homo Sacer* is a life which in itself interests the *polis* 'objectively', but which from a subjective point of view is a matter of indifference. *Homo Sacer* stands for the other as less than citizen and less than slave or woman. *Homo Sacer* is presumed capable of suffering the effects of law but not of enjoying its protection; as if he or she 'can suffer' but 'cannot affect' anyone.[5] In sum, Orestes can be said to have

---

[5]Going back to my earlier discussions, Agamben's modern individual can be understood as the *Sidaway* woman (who, as we saw in Chapter 4, is protected by the law only as object of therapeutic medical decision-making) or, even more clearly, as the *Bland* man (see Chapter 1). As we saw in the analysis of the *Bland* case, whether the indeterminate

been the exceptional being whom the political-juridical order of Argos 'included through exclusion' and whom it identified purely as object and not as self-identical unique being. In Agamben's terms, Orestes' 'naked life' would be the object of 'abandonment'; in my terms his 'useless' suffering becomes the 'non-object' of civil indifference. In this Greek example, moreover, I show that that which Agamben called 'gradual' process of politicisation of 'naked life' from Roman times to modernity was, already in *Eumenides,* a story foretold. I believe that Aeschylus refers to the pre-classical harsh Argosian laws institution just as Agamben looks at *Homo Sacer.* And, just as in Agamben's view of late modernity, Aeschylus adds a twist to Orestes' story whereby Orestes is later received by the city of Athens.

It is important to note that the 'first' Athenian criminal trial ever was one that, possibly, ought not to have happened at all - according to the law. Orestes had, through his horrendous deed, not so much 'violated the law' as become half-human, at the margin of civilisation, a subject of difference but of no identity. He was of interest to the law only as subjectivity in exile, 'included-as-excluded'. On what account could the Athenian court turn towards the case of polluted Orestes in the first place? How is it that law's agents can change from being indifferent towards the subjectivity in exile to being interested in identifying Orestes as criminal, seeking out his origins and evidence of guilt or innocence? In short, prior to there being a legal case to contest, the 'central' issue in *Eumenides* is the very subjective *admissibility* of Orestes, the subject of 'indifferent difference', in the Athenian justice system. This is not merely a question of 'natural' justice and giving the suspect a 'fair trial'. One must not underestimate the fact that for Aeschylus the trial in question was not just 'a trial' but the 'first trial' ever. Rather, I argue, an 'unnatural' justice was offered to Orestes and interrupted his exile. It is a question of justice being born to obsessive approach and charity offered by the subjects of Athenian and divine laws to the almost inhuman subject-in-exile who did not 'deserve' fairness. The question of polluted Orestes' admissibility to Athenian society was not answered by the arguments of Apollo and Athena, which are addressing the 'secondary' issue of Orestes innocence or

---

vegetating other is defined in terms of material immanent interests or abstract 'transcendent' juridical rights is theoretically of no great importance. Both the medical idea of the other's 'interest' and the juridical one of the other's 'right' would be explained by Agamben in similar terms under his extended view of biopolitics. As we saw, the law on the vegetating that the case involves excludes mortality and rather discusses issues of quality of life. But this law must not be studied only as if articulating the 'passage' between the natural life of the a-conscious living thing which ignores its social surroundings and the 'proper' political existence of being in language and consciousness. As Agamben helps us to understand, the 'politicisation' of Bland's *zoe* or 'naked life' that this 'quality of life' decision entails and in which the patient's factual interests were blurred with abstract rights, rests on particular kind of *apprehension* of his whole being which combines the order of sovereign rights and that of biopolitical interests.

guilt. Moreover, those arguments 'in Orestes' defence' are ultimately more about the self-interest of those who make them: Apollo and Athena use Orestes' case in order to usurp jurisdiction from the Furies - goddesses of fury and guilt. Apollo announces that Orestes had already been purified in Delphi by himself, albeit he was not competent to purify criminals (only the Furies could do so). Athena opts for persuasion, claiming that matricide is less polluting than parricide. These individual interests were not sufficient reasons for the Athenian citizens to lose their fear of approaching the stranger. The reason, therefore, has to be sought elsewhere.

At this point, and prior to any argument, I must emphasise that I want to avoid an easily made assumption about Aeschylus' play; namely, that the story revolves around the moment of 'transition' from consuetudinary or chthonic religious law to 'formal' secular Greek law, as is the case in the more famous Greek tragedy *Antigone*. From our modern standpoint it is easy to think that Aeschylus' trilogy, too, narrates 'progressively' how 'formal law', represented by the law of Athens, succeeded in superseding the ancestral and chthonic laws, represented by the Furies. One is tempted to think this because in the play the Furies are depicted as the victims of cunning persuasion by the 'new gods' Apollo and Athena, who stand for human law and who take the side of Orestes - apparently from self-interested 'philanthropy' in the case of Apollo and from misogynist self-hatred in the case of the goddess Athena. Athena's main legal argument is that the slaughter of a mother is 'less grave' than parricide, so that the slaughter of Clytaemnestra by her son deserved a less severe revenge than the one she incurred by slaying her husband. At the end of the play the Furies discover they have been 'cheated' out of their jurisdiction by the new gods' rhetoric, and promise to keep returning to Athens bringing catastrophe. But even if the trilogy is thus seen as if consisting of progressive stages of the triumph of formal law over old law, culminating in the self-interested advocacy of the gods in the last part of the final play, still it seems to suggest a lesson. Formal law, that is, cannot really 'supersede' but only incorporate the force of 'ancestral' law, which is used by some writers as a metaphor for ethical action.

Indeed, one major theme of Aeschylus' trilogy is the ambiguous notion of *Dike,* the cosmic principle of justice that governs the dealings of gods and mortals, and whose dictates man ignores at his peril (Podlecki 1984: 63). As well as representing a metaphysical concept the term also denoted the *concrete proceedings-at-law* to which the Greeks of the time of Aeschylus (and before) had recourse. My assumption is that Aeschylus' trilogy can be seen as a dramatic whole which preserves this unity of *Dike.* After all, at the very end of the story the Furies are not 'transformed' into Eumenides - the play merely reveals that the Furies (symbols of eternal persecution and guilt) are *also* to be known as Eumenides (obsessed with the good, wildly charitable). It is only if the three plays are presented 'in progression' towards a concluding *telos* that the unity of law and justice, Furies and Eumenides in it lapses. But let me perform a different reading of the myth and use it to show how all kinds of justice (formalised or otherwise) are inseparable from and unthinkable without charity. However, if Orestes exemplifies the tentative relation of interest/indifference that the *polis* maintains with the 'naked being' as abstract legal subject, we need a third standpoint to add to those of interest and indifference, perhaps that of disinterestedness, in relation to which we can explain law's opening to the other *as other*. Such a principle may be traced in the following pleadings by Orestes which address the question of his being 'already' cleansed and therefore approachable. Once in Athens, Orestes begins his plea with reference to a prior 'purification' which stems directly from human proximity (rather than the false one that Apollo had performed):

> A suppliant in need of purification I am not ... and do thou of thy grace receive an accursed wretch, no suppliant for purification, or uncleansed of hand, but with my guilt's edge already blunted and worn away at other habitations and in the travelled paths of men ... I now approach thy house ... [H]ere will I keep my post and abide the issue of my trial (at 235-241);

and:

> It [would be] a long tale to tell from the beginning of all I visited and harmed not by my dwelling with them (276-286).

Several aspects of this plea must be emphasised. First, Orestes' does not make reference to Apollo's purificatory ritual. Orestes' words thus upset any presumption that his admissibility to court rested on his divine purification by the power-seeking new gods of 'legal' justice. For that purification had no validity in being an unwarranted use of ritual, and itself needing justification. Could it be, as I think, that legal justice is born to disinterested charity? Interestingly, Orestes' plea emphasises that whilst in exile he had been received by many 'others' and that he had travelled, not as a wild animal but 'in the travelled paths of men'. It is indeed remarkable that the destitute Orestes, standing at the 'gates' of Athenian society, begins his plea *not* by recounting the suffering he had incurred in his long wanderings in order to plead for empathic or sympathetic mercy, but with a reference to the charitable hospitality he had had the chance to *enjoy*, as if his enjoyment of proximity had in itself already 'cleansed' him of the pollution of being eternally rejected, and had 'rubbed it off' on the others whom he met, who thus became responsible for his crimes!

'How', one may ask, 'was Orestes capable of enjoyment while in exile in the first place? Indeed, enjoyment presupposes self-identical subjectivity and individuation, while the 'subjectivity-in-exile', as I have defined it, lacks individuation. Perhaps one must suppose that the pre-original source of human individuation lies in the charity and gratuitousness of human approach. Disinterested approach governs proximity with the otherwise than being (which the vulnerable stranger represents), operating independently of whether he or she *is/is not* included in the inter-*esse* of the *polis*. Finally, we must enquire into the motives and *responsibility of those who offered purificatory but also 'excessive' hospitality* to Orestes. Could it be the result of knowledge of and/or mimetic desire for what Orestes' being 'was' and 'had'? If so, then it would have been a knowledge of/desire for 'subjectivity-in-exile' - i.e. that which is a different living entity but not a self-same individual. The Greek duty of philoxenia excluded unwanted strangers such as the 'polluted'; indeed anyone who came into proximity with the 'polluted' became polluted himself, thus becoming incapable of 'cleansing' anyone else. In consequence, the hospitality offered to Orestes exceeded a relationship based on knowledge and desire and is evidence of an anarchic 'one-way' moral obligation to welcome the other which by far surpasses the notions of duty and reciprocal obligation. Alternatively, could it perhaps be that Orestes' plea invokes merely 'accidental' encounters and hospitality rather than hospitality which was willingly extended to him by his hosts? Was there freedom and judgement? Was the hospitality given voluntarily ? In short, are the hosts *responsible* for purifying *contra lege* and *contra natura* law's first client? If there was responsibility there must have been judgement. Yet, if this was in the form of inescapable moral obligation (to say 'yes' first, then judge) we must look beyond 'objective' or 'subjective' judgement, beyond choice and intentionality. We must look for traces of 'counter-intentional judg(e)ment'.

I submit that the question of Orestes' admissibility to Athenian society - prior to that of his 'fair' or 'unfair' trial - concerns the judg(e)ment made by the Athenians who listened to his plea concerning his, ultimately, *absurd* suffering which does not enter into the equation *hubris*-fate. No proper reason was offered for deciding to approach the stranger; indeed 'deciding' is a strong word for what was an involuntary act of charity. It was the charity of interrogating the other's suffering without any interest, fear or repulsion that effectively 'cleansed' Orestes. At issue is not merely the admissibility of Orestes in the inter-*esse* of legal subjects in Athens but their *approaching him*. We cannot subsume this problem under a model of transformation or conversion from legal 'indifference' into bio-political 'interest'. It is rather that, paradoxically, the alternatives of interest and indifference require a residual, inexhaustible disinterestedness towards the other. However, *who* does it take to recognise the 'otherwise than being'? And how does it feel to feel free to approach the subjectivity-in-exile, despite its horrific suffering, rather than to keep away from the 'impurity' of its non-sensical fate? The author of *Eumenides* has not attempted in his story to identify those hosts of Orestes who, by offering him proximity, 'purified' him and allowed him later to enter Athens. I argue that the originary 'purificatory' event of anarchic donation of *philoxenia* towards the 'naked' other must not be attributed to accident or be seen as mistaken application of customary rules of hospitality.

The judg(e)ment on absurd suffering is not a misjudgement. Nor is it pertinent to ask whether Orestes acquired his hosts' proximity by fraud and misrepresentation of his situation as fugitive. (In any case Orestes' poor appearance before his hosts, after a long period of wandering, would certainly have betrayed his secret.) But, these are not appropriate questions to ask. It is not important whether the other suffers by mistake or fault. The destitution and suffering of the other human cannot be apprehended nor comprehended by me. The other's suffering signifies to *me* a demand for infinite charity, whilst it does not promise me delivery from the feeling of guilt. *My* guilt and responsibility is the *only* meaning that attaches to the event of coming across my other's sufferings. Beyond this meaning of the me-for-the-other the other's destitution constitutes only absurd and useless suffering. The charitable act of hospitality, which makes law possible, is not a response to a duty but the experience of moral obligation.

It cannot be stressed enough that Lévinas' accounts of 'moral obligation' constitute a search for the original significance of an *unmediated* experience of obligation and as such is very different from the obedience to law in Kant. Obligation is an 'order having its authority in itself' and does not need a universal place - *'neutre'*, *arche* or Being - to acquire its meaning and its power to bind a subject. Like suffering it subjects the subject to a counter-experience. Aeschylus' dramatic transmission of the myth of the origins of justice includes - perhaps unintentionally - a *prophecy:* the universal meaning of subjectivity will not ever become transformed fully into obedience to the law. However, I have argued, subjectivity can be understood as excessive responsibility for the other's suffering which is less than the 'object' of intentionality and more than the 'non-object' of indifference; nor is 'ethical subjectivity' to be equated with 'psychological content'. The experience of being-for-the-other is, rather, made up of pure emotion which occurs for nothing: it is affectivity beyond experience. That which is universal in this case is the obligation to endure being the hostage of my neighbour. Before the vulnerable other, the other as otherwise than being/non-being, the self is faced with a universal obligation; but due to the excesses of its responsibility the subjectivity cannot match this experience of obligation with knowledge or desire. Therefore, although the obligation to be-for-the-other is universal it concerns me and my other exclusively in so far as I am unaware of universality. A 'unique' other 'for me and my responsibility' is (obsessively) desired by me. Thus stripped of sovereignty, my self approaches the other as 'the only one that matters for me'- without question. In so doing the self marks the other with an *identity of uniqueness* to match its all-important difference as 'exiled', vulnerable subjectivity.

III
Ethical proximity in the ethics of alterity and the 'aporia' of justice

Thomas Keenan has recently attempted to tie Lévinas' notion of subjectivity as 'hostage' of the other with the so-called 'aporetic politics of justice' (Keenan

1997: 7-42). Before looking at his argument let me reiterate how I understand the notion of subjectivity as 'hostage'. The word 'I' means *here I am*, answering for everything and everyone. It requires subjectivity 'in the accusative' and a self which must exist, as I have termed it earlier, 'despite itself' in suffering responsibility for another. Moved by its guilt for not being able to die in its other's place, 'this self is out of phase with itself, by itself [*Soi déphasé par soi*]', originally ruptured and exposed by 'the force of an alterity in it' (AE: 114-15). The adventure of subjectivity with its other begins thus in the disinterested relation to otherness, or else, in 'exile' from inter-*esse*. One's non-sensical suffering must become another's consciousness and sense of one's own responsibility. 'To be oneself, the state of being a hostage, [is] always to have one *degree* of responsibility more, the responsibility for the responsibility of the other' (AE: 117). This higher 'degree' of responsibility is desired by the self who approaches the destitute other as the 'only one that matters', stripped of characteristics, self-coincidence and interests, yet significant. As we saw in Chapter 2, it is with this abstract yet unique other that the liberal discourse seems to be obsessed in declaring the existence of *a-priori* human rights whereby the other human is 'extracted' from all reference to his or her 'natural' or sociological circumstances.

On these premises Keenan constructs an argument on the possibility of 'justice' being realised by the subject's decisions and actions. He argues that the question whether actual justice is possible must be continuously recast and remain open 'if we are to give justice its due' (Keenan 1997: 28). This view is compatible with the one I have been taking whereby coming across the indeterminacy (or, 'aporia') of justice requires a personal and irrepressibly surprising emotional adventure and restlessness of the self as the unique subjectivity for the other that belies the judging 'I'. Any so-called 'impersonal' or 'neutral judgment' (customarily spelled without the 'e' in the case of juridical decision) is also found to be an inescapably personal one, or a judg(e)ment. For me, moreover, even that second, 'subjective' aspect of the judgement - which refers to the judge's *psyche* - that is, the 'dialogue of the soul with itself' - does not yet reveal the most intimate secret of the judging subjectivity. The latter is to be found on the counter-intentional *affective* impact of the judged other on the judge's subjectivity, which reveals the judge to be a subject of responsibility as proximity, engaged through disengagement with the human beings whose dispute he or she is adjudicating. That is, 'to judge' is first of all to act out of obsession (not compulsion) and charity and to come to engage 'disinterestedly' with others; that is, to approach them otherwise than in terms of subjective/objective memory and representation, i.e. as 'naked' subjectivities in exile, hovering between being and non-being, essence and inessence, presence and absence calling for approach beyond inter-*esse*. Absurd as it may appear, it is thus that I must 'face' each of my others before I am able to proffer 'judgment' in which my subjectivity disappears, substituted by my subjective/objective views of the others that I judge or am judged by.

To many progressive thinkers, however, the above views on the 'impossibility' of actual justice appear restrictive, if not quietist. As Keenan says, many assume that 'because justice is possible, but not actual, action is called forth to bring it out of the taunting ideality of the potential into reality' (Keenan 1997: 29). Thus, for the deconstructionist the crucial question remains:

> [W]hat might deconstruction ... have to contribute to the question of the impossibility of justice? ... The claim that deconstruction could contribute something to the question of justice, possible or impossible, comes these days as either self-evident or an outrage (and hence, in both cases as unthought). More than a quarter of a century after *De la Grammatologie* ... and a decade after *Allegories of Reading*, academic ... commonplaces remain unaccountably but desperately impoverished in their encounters with the question (ibid. 29-30).[6]

Keenan comes very close to the Derridean thesis on the 'impossibility of justice'. In this regard it is worth remembering that although Derrida's minimalistic view of justice as *command* is close to that of Lévinas, the two differ in that Lévinas emphasises the passivity of the singular subject of moral experience, whilst Derrida focuses on the force of the universal command. In consequence, whilst Lévinas' philosophy is spent trying to express that the experience of being commanded to be moral 'for nothing' is *unique*, and that to be 'just' means risking oneself in the *anarchy* of compassion and charity, deconstruction sets itself different aims:

> How are we to *distinguish* between the force of law of a legitimate power and the supposedly originary violence that must have established this authority and that could not itself have been authorised by any anterior legitimacy, so that, in this initial moment, it is neither legal nor illegal ... neither just nor unjust? (Derrida in Rosenfeld ed. 1992: 6; my emphasis).

The 'supposition' of originary violence would not trouble Lévinas whose ineluctable 'violence of compassion' is not an 'originary act' which precedes and founds authority but a 'pre-original' and 'diachronic' pre-requisite for justice. Keenan understands well that 'Lévinas' hostage is [a being caught] between autonomy and submission to an imperative ... [and] this subject thrives on its own

---

[6]And further, 'Deconstruction's ethico-political pertinence is either (i) taken for granted ... with an appeal to its thematic or referential consideration of issues (democracy, torture, feminism, the university and teaching, apartheid) or to its formal homologies with political interventions (deconstruction of authority as emancipatory or ideology-critique), or (ii) condemned (as anti-political or paralysing) because it appears to ruin the categories on which political discourse has tried to found itself for as long as it can remember: subjectivity and agency, and the reliable knowledge (meaning--whether positively, theologically, or hermeneutically determined) that seems to ground its action' (Keenan 1997: 29).

scission' - although I am not so sure that 'thrives' is the right word (Keenan 1997: 31). It is for this reason that my 'Lévinasian' justice-model (which I have employed throughout in my analysis of legal cases) focuses on 'responsibility' rather than 'content' of decisions and actions. Whether the 'content' is 'just' or 'unjust' depends on whether or not it is surrounded by responsibility. This raises the issue of justification which is deconstruction's central problem too. In this connection I submit that Keenan sides with the 'aporetic' rather than the 'ethical' view of justice. To illustrate, let me follow Keenan's critique of Fish. Keenan reviews the position of Stanley Fish in his 'Force', which contains his consideration of the deconstructionist 'quest for quarantining the process of law from force', a quest which is 'doomed by definition to failure' because law is unthinkable without rhetoric, and '[R]hetoric is another word for force' (Keenan 1997: 16). As Keenan observes, Fish engages with the notion of a 'psychological core' which is arguably shared by thinkers as disparate as H. L. A. Hart and Terry Eagleton. 'Eagleton', Fish reports, 'equates being *forced mindlessly* into an action by an ideological obsession with the pressure of somebody holding a gun to my head' (ibid. 16). The term 'ideological obsession' connotes an:

> ideological misrecognition that empties the mind by filling it with what belongs outside. [An] ... error ... that of metonymic reversal: what should be outside, too close for comfort but nevertheless still alien, changes places, comes to hollow out what it threatened and substitute itself for its victim (ibid. 17).

In this connection, Fish argues in 'Force' that the metaphor of inside/outside '(what Paul de Man once memorably called a "binary polarity of classical banality in the history of metaphysics")', which lends itself so well to these reversals, is itself aberrant: there is no difference between the mind, the psychological core of rationality, and all those dangerous prejudices and coercions that apparently threaten it - without them, you are nothing. These obsessions, whether we call them beliefs or fashions or biases or interests, are the very condition in and on which we 'calculate, determine, and decide' (ibid. 17). Indeed, Fish writes that 'a mind divested of all direction could not recognise any reason for going in one direction at all' (ibid.). But also, that to 'free your mind' of its obsessions would then amount to 'freeing your mind of itself, to rendering yourself mindless' (ibid.). Moreover, he concludes:

> the force of law is always and already indistinguishable from the forces it would oppose ... There is always a gun at your head. Sometimes the gun is, in literal fact, a gun; sometimes it is as a reason, an assertion whose weight is inseparable from some already assumed purpose; sometimes it is a desire, the urging of a state of affairs to which you are already predisposed; sometimes it is a need you already feel; sometimes it is a name - country, justice, honour, love, God - whose power you have already internalised (ibid.).

Keenan makes some very insightful observations on Fish's position and points to how Fish begins his argument with the motif of compulsion and force but ends, for no apparent reason (Keenan says, 'mechanism unknown') with a standard metaphysical definition of the subject as self-compelled. He says, including quotes from Fish, that:

> Fish's argument risks the temptation to replace the deconstructed polarity of inside/outside, gun up against head, with an almost-admitted monism: if the critical distance offered by the binary model is untenable and resistance to the call of the other (heteronomy) impossible - if 'this is precisely what one cannot possibly do and still remain a 'one', a being with a capacity for action' - then you can never get away from yourself, from your one self, 'from the pressure exerted by a partial, non-neutral, non authoritative, ungrounded point of view' (519) that makes you the you that you are (Kenenan 1997: 17).

Keenan shows how Fish puts all the emphasis 'on stasis' and so stasis preserves:

> the classical condition of decisive action, the subject's upright stance before the object, the subject of *Vorstellung* as, in Fish's own words, 'a one, a being with a capacity for action' (ibid. 18).

In terms of Lévinas' discourse, I submit that what Fish is interested to depict here, which annoyed Keenan, is the work of *essence* in the subject of consciousness. As I pointed out earlier, Lévinas describes 'essence' (or, *conatus*) as the active persistence of being in 'being-for-itself' or, an 'invincible persistence in essence, filling up every interval of nothingness which would interrupt its exercise' (AE: 4). Consciousness *ignores* its counter-affectivity and is blind to how its obsessions transcend the false dilemma 'freedom from external force' or 'radical irresponsibility'. It assumes that it can either persist in essence or 'die'. That is, it is assumed that consciousness cannot take leave of itself, say 'adieu' and face infinity without being shattered, surviving, as it were, by means of an ethical miracle. Inertia is the result of persistence in one's internalised beliefs, fashions, biases, interests; the very condition in and on which we calculate, determine, and decide, that without which the subject would 'lose its mind'. Fish's consciousness is arrested in fear before a false dilemma. He seems caught between assuming the otherness he encounters through the work of collection, presentation and interpretation of phenomenality, or *dying* because the encounter with exteriority-as-alterity deals the self-closure of the subject of consciousness a 'fatal' blow. In all this we hear the echo of the slogan 'individual freedom or death' which has been adopted by most modern western liberal revolutions. It is in this way that consciousness, fearful of the otherness of death, posits its own limitations in how far it will undergo an opening-up to otherness. Delimited consciousness supposedly does not have the time to be moved excessively by the other: it rather dwells on its pleasant or unpleasant experiences before something or someone puts it out of existence. Time's patience as *dureé* leaves unaffected this vigilant and self-preoccupied consciousness which is allergic to otherness. In this regard Keenan accuses Fish's model of speaking about the 'subject of *Vorstellung*'. This is the subject which, even in 'stasis' and inertia, is said to retain the capacity to decide and act. But, in this way, consciousness is thought of as bereft of what Lévinas calls the 'miracle' whereby consciousness is shocked to encounter in the other the idea of infinity *without*, however, being destroyed as a result. In this light, I disagree with Keenan's decision to continue Fish's metaphor of the other as a 'gun pressed against one's head':

> there must be a gun ... The gun figures not simply force, the distorting effects of what is not properly mine, but necessity, the stark and non-negotiable demand to submit, which can only be exercised by the other (Keenan 1997: 41).

To be sure, Lévinas insists on the dis-propriating effect of the address, the appeal, or the pressure to which I am subjected, and on the contradictory burdens it puts on the one who must respond. Indeed, a responsibility for the other which has not begun in me, appears responsibility in 'innocence' - the innocence of being hostage. However, although my responsibility for another is *not* my choice, *nor* is it an 'accident' that happened to me, it is responsibility for the other that will not return to myself, signifying 'selfhood' without virility, as exasperated contracting which cannot be contained from within the limits of self-identity. This responsibility for another is an insatiable charity which does not measure in the same way as the subject's freedom to 'assume' or 'decline' responsibility. Indeed, my responsibility has not awaited my freedom in which a commitment to my other would have already been decided by me; it is a 'force' which 'precedes' my contraction and essence. I have not implicated myself with the other and yet I am 'under accusation' for his or her sake by the universal moral command to be-for-my-other: I am, in a way, 'persecuted'. In terms of law, Keenan says, with reference to Derrida, the 'persecution' of the subject corresponds to a double command: to be ethical and just at once. This, for him, constitutes an 'enigma'. Thus, ethics:

> is the force essentially implied in the concept of *justice as law (droit)* [which makes Derrida insist on reserving the possibility of] a justice ... that not only exceeds or contradicts 'law' (*droit*) but also, perhaps, has no relation to law, or maintains such a strange relation to it that it may just as well command the '*droit*' that excludes it ... Enigma: what is it that '... exceeds or contradicts law', but also '... has no relationship to law'? (Keenan 1997: 5).

Answer: such 'force' as Derrida and Keenan attempt to describe cannot be presented in universal terms - it must, however, be assumed. First, its description is linked always with particular subjects of excessive obligations and emotions.

Second, at best, it can be universalised as a *mode* of being, in particular a *dés-intér-essement* which is not indifference, but obsession and charity, which prevent the subject from complacency and indifference. 'Justice' *is* to *be there for the other*. Derrida says that indeed justice as thematisation and calculation is paradoxically linked to 'gift', beyond exchange and distribution, the undecidable, the incommensurable or the incalculable, i.e. singularity, difference and heterogeneity (Derrida 1992, 1995). But he withholds from us the gift of *his* responsibility when in what follows he implicitly 'exempts' risk from responsibility: 'one cannot speak directly about justice, thematise or objectivise justice, say 'this is just' and even less 'I am just', without immediately betraying justice' (Derrida 1992: 10). The difference between deconstructionist ethics and ethics as *prima philosophia* is as follows. In Keenan's phrase 'the address, the appeal, or the pressure to which I am subjected, and on the contradictory burdens it puts on the one who must respond', the emphasis is on the address, appeal or pressure which *addresses anyone,* and not, as it would be in Lévinas, on the individuated way in which each subject suffers its responsibility, in a unique manner.[7] In short, Keenan is keen to adopt a position whereby in spite of the fact that the other's demand 'freezes' the self into an inwardness, an intimity or stasis, the self is ultimately 'replaceable' because 'it could be anyone' who responds. This position on subjectivity as 'happenstance' ties in with Blanchot's notion of 'disindividuation' (*désindividuation*). Blanchot wrote:

> In the patience of passivity, I am he whom anyone at all can replace ... but one for whom nonetheless there is no dispensation: he must answer to and for what he is not (Blanchot 1986: 35).

Notice how the emphasis on the subject's responsibility 'for what he is not' distracts from what I have called the oscillation and restlessness of self, that is its emotiveness and exposure when it is moved 'beyond measure' by the other. In relation to Blanchot's disparity with Lévinas, which is at issue here, Fabio Ciaramelli has charged Blanchot with 'distort[ing] radically Lévinas' understanding of the hostage's condition (or uncondition)' (Bernasconi 1991: 105 n. 76). Indeed, in Lévinas the self is obsessed that, in response to the call of the other for help, he or she is the *only* responsible one: It asks itself – 'if not me then who else?'. For Lévinas without this *self-assignation/persecution* there can be unicity in the self; my own responsibility becomes the only valid *principium*

---

[7]Keenan sums up his views:
'It happens every day ... - on the street, on television, from passer-by, friends and relatives, world leaders - and it singles us out in a peculiar way. There is cry for help, addressed not to me, but to me as anyone - anyone can help - and my anonymity in this situation, far from offering an excuse to ignore the plea, implicates me directly. Not because I know anything or because of my 'already'-existing desires and interests, but because *I happen to be there*' (Keenan 1997: 23; my emphasis).

individuationis. Yet this utterly individuated *me* also obeys a universal ethical demand. 'Universality' concerns the other's demand or appeal: indeed, as Keenan says, the other who cries is calling out to 'anyone'. Vulnerability and suffering constitute the knot of humanity. By contrast, as Ciaramelli has correctly pointed out, Blanchot introduces a *theatrical* element which does not suit Lévinas' view of proximity:

> the radicality of [Levinas' proximity] demands that we conceive proximity to exclude the possibility of theatre: 'le rôle du moi' is mine alone and no one can play this part except me (Ciaramelli in Bernasconi 1991: 99).

Yet, for Keenan, Blanchot 'radicalises what remains hesitant in Lévinas: *assignation irrécusable*, yes, singular address, but not exactly to 'me' or to my subjected self' (Keenan 1997: 21). In this regard, I strongly disagree with Blanchot and Keenan and must side with Ciaramelli. The question 'am I replaceable or not before my other' is a question for *me*. To put it in terms of Aeschylus' myth, the people who offered unconditional hospitality to Orestes (thus preparing him for the court) and the court in Athens could, of course, have been 'anyone', but the burden had already been assumed by *them*. Also, Keenan's argument implies that 'there is' a subject which faces 'contradictory pressures', a subject of 'dilemmas'. The contradiction concerns the 'multiple demands' others make on me. It is my argument that this is much less a radical view of subjectivity than the one which says that the contradiction concerns the *attitudes* which the subject incarnates in relation to those demands: this critically varies from *disinterested approach* to *interest* and, finally, *indifference*. In terms of disinterestedness the question of 'who is' the addressee of the universal command 'be for each other' is not yet posed.

In all, Keenan and Blanchot differ from Lévinas in (i) equating (and so underplaying) the universality of the demand with its multiple manifestations by my different others, and (ii) assuming that because the other cries out 'to anyone', this means that I must, reciprocally, respond to my other '*as* anyone'. Keenan, thus, equally with Blanchot, distorts Lévinas' thesis that an utterly individuated me obeys a universal demand. For *me* there is no question of universality or reciprocity with regard to my self's disinterested, yet obsessive, assumption of responsibility for my neighbour. I am individuated (i) in my astonishment before the infinite vulnerability of my other - a vulnerability that exceeds the pair subject-object - I do not care if his/her appeal is addressed to 'anyone' or 'someone' and; therefore, the question whether I am facing the obligation to help as 'someone' or 'anyone' is not yet posed. 'Me' is all-important to the other but not because of my difference and identity: I am subjectivity which matters to the other but I am also stripped of self-identity. In consequence, I become obsessed that, for the purpose of helping the other, I am *the one* rather than either 'someone' or 'anyone'. And (ii) I am individuated by means of my own 'one-way actions' which direct towards the other my desire to join and enjoy him or her as *unique* other, as otherwise than being/having; this is the meaning of my claiming the other human to be the subject of high rights. My 'inwardness' is in fact constituted by this reference to my unique other which is anarchical, indiscreet towards otherness and characterised by the 'violence of the good' (in the sense I gave in Chapter 2). On a *prophetic* level, Aeschylus' story above proposes Orestes as the subjectivity in exile which *obsesses* all his hosts, including his Athenian judges.

IV
The Messiah is *me*

Lévinas' description of ethical subjectivity as the 'elected one' is inseparable from prophecy. Is not his 'charitable subject of justice' bound always to put itself (psychotically?) in the place of the Messiah for the sake of its others? As C. Chalier has pointed out, there is a crucial link between Lévinas' thinking of ipseity (i.e. the singular subjectivity of a universal morality) and messianism (C. Chalier in Rolland ed. 1984). Further, F. Ciaramelli suggests that:

> The election of the subject is thought of in the light of Israel, which is only an election in the sense of a *'charge écrasante'* that one has to bear. Such an election is, in Lévinas' words, 'no doubt a *malheur'*. The parallel holds provided we recognise that *despite* its insurmountable particularity, Israel's election has, just as in the case of the individual, a meaning that is universal and which concerns the whole of humanity. Each and every person is called upon to *accomplish* this *'destinée'* which shows itself in the history and spirituality of Hebraism. For the ethical subject, prophetic testimony of one's own election is the inspired Saying of the ethical vocation of humanity (Ciaramelli in Bernasconi and Critchley eds. 1991: 98-99).

And:

> Ultimately, the same issue [i.e. of ipseity: being oneself as 'the one' for the other:] is at stake in Lévinas' meditation on Jewish messianism and its difference from the Christian identification of the Messiah in the person of Jesus. 'Hebraism would announce a form of existence beyond the individual Messiah, whose individuation is not realised in a single being.' All peoples are the Messiah to the extent that they become a me, responsible for others. *'The Messiah is me. To be Me is to be the Messiah'*... (op. cit. 99-101). [8]

---

[8]As such, 'prophetic testimony cannot be objective in character, for this would be to gather transcendence into the universality of the *logos*. And neither can it be a confession of an inner condition or conviction, for then transcendence would be a matter of empirical

In the first of the two quotations above I have italicised the word 'despite' in order to emphasise that, in ethical responsibility, the subject assumes its destined 'oneness' *despite itself.* The words 'accomplish this destiny', too, must be understood neither in terms of freedom of choice *nor* of compulsion, but instead, in terms of messianic obsession and the radical freedom it brings. The story of Orestes that I told earlier and the Hebrew teachings share a universal morality; they both assume a subject of unique difference but not self-same identity as the common pre-origin of charity and justice. However, only the Greek story, a story for theatre set long before the advent in Greece of Christianity and Neoplatonism, uses the singular figure of the destitute individual in exile in order to 'found' legal institutions. In other words, this Greek myth and history can express the uniquely different but not self-identical subjectivity only as subjectivity 'in exile', whereby the other is of interest to the *polis.* The narrative is acted (and *said*) in the *polis for* the *polis* - its purposes and ideology constitute its subject. The plot is only partly interested in Orestes; of interest is the guest Athens brought in - who could make reasonable arguments in his defence. But, if spoken by Hebraic lips - in a synagogue, where to 'speak' is to 'pray' or to 'turn towards the Highest'- the same pagan story would sound different. Then, 'exile' concerns *people* and *humanity* rather than the 'individual' and the 'city'. The important element in Orestes' story would not be the relationship of Orestes with the *polis* that rejected him and the one that later admitted him, but rather his uninterrupted *humanity* during exile. This expresses how the *singular* inessential ethical subject relates to the *universal* 'ethical vocation of humanity' (see Chalier above) through its 'useless suffering' and excessive acts of charity. As Ciaramelli writes (above), in Lévinas the ethical subject witnesses suffering and prophesies its own election as Messiah. Moreover, the story shows that the city cannot deny the disinterestedness which precedes and makes possible its laws which bring symmetry to antagonism and maintain the peace of inter-*esse.* Thus, from a Hebraic 'prophetic' perspective, the story of Orestes is read as conveying a lesson: that justice is inseparable from charity.

Again, it must be stressed that this *messianic* approach proximity is maintained only if we understand fully what 'accomplishing' a destiny *despite* one's intentions means. 'Counter-intentional obsession' is necessary in order that the ethical subject does not ever manage to declare itself universal and of absolute value simply because it is 'dealt' a universal moral obligation. The relationship between individuation and universality is one of radically asymmetrical responsibility of the one for the other. In these conditions the 'ethical freedom' of subjectivity must be understood as *disinterestedness* or, as Ciaramelli writes: 'the liberation from ontological necessities and cares, a refusal of the *conatus essendi* and a deliverance from being'. In Lévinas' terms, the freedom and power to 'accomplish' moral destiny 'signify the *acceptance* of a vocation to which I alone

---

psychology. No, it is the simple statement of a truth, neither anonymous nor neutral, but entirely personal and even ideologically pure' (ibid.).

can respond, or again, the power to respond to [the vocation] when called. To be free is only to do what nobody else can do in my place' (ADV 1982: 178 n. 6). In fact '[T]he absolute and disinterested generosity of responsibility implies ... a radical individuation transcending ... [all] generality or the generalising power of death. However, by no means does this signify a search for immortality. On the contrary, it calls upon the subject to refrain from assisting in the accomplishment of his or her own actions. In such a radical passivity or patience, subjectivity is being-for-beyond-my-death'.

A more general implication from comparison of the view of ethical responsibility as being 'hostage' in, respectively, Lévinas's purely philosophical discourse and Derrida's 'aporetic justice', is that ethical subjectivity in the latter is, in the end, deemed marginal, exceptional, fleeting, much as in ontological discourse. Therefore the political inferences deconstructionists draw from Lévinas' idea of 'hostage' are not yet as radical as they need to be to tackle the ontological politics which reduce the vocation of compassion to a mere psychological symptom. We saw this reduction in *Bland* where the relation of the judges to the other is understood in law as an 'activity' (as is also the case, as I have shown, in theories such as those of Cornell and Fish). The active, conscious subject is assumed to triumph after a period of only seeming (temporary) passivity before otherness. By means of memory and interpretation the interested, essentially active subject of consciousness takes the temporal dispersion, and all events that occurred in it, back into itself. But thinking is necessarily remembrance, and thought is recollection. The order of being and of society which the focus on activity establishes is an eternal return of the same. Thus consciousness of the being-for-the-other becomes an 'eon' and reverts to 'being-for-itself', dwelling excessively on its limited power to imagine or (alternatively) ignore the other. The being-for-the-other which the proximity to the neighbour in alterity entails becomes unaccountable because of its radical passivity, which is not translatable into the categories of free will. In these circumstances 'responsibility' continues to appear meaningless and absurd if it does not follow 'free choice', that is, if it is without the force that makes it an object of a free assumption and voluntary taking on of a charge. Thus, the 'subject' is always thought of as if capable of matching the force of responsibility for the absurd sufferings of its other by means of an self-generated 'own' force: be it through knowledge or desire or some kind of empathy. And, in consequence, the absurdity of the suffering of one's other can no longer be recognised because my intentionality has apprehended it; it can now even be the object of judgment, and, at the same time, it entails only a limited responsibility on my side, that supposedly can be sufficiently heeded.

What enables the subject of consciousness to revert from being responsible 'for nothing' to being-responsible-for-itself? There is a force that the subject must never lose if it is to be recognised as ineluctably social ('political'). Agamben talks of how being's 'naked' life (*zoe*) becomes political life (*bios*) through the 'power to speak of itself' before all third others. This power is an essential precondition for self-accounting. For Agamben, further, human socialisation requires this power in the form of language, and abandonment of one's 'nakedness' to the interest/indifference of the *polis*:

> the living animal possesses *logos* by suppressing and conserving in itself its own voice just as he inhabits the *polis* by letting his naked life be exempted in it (Agamben 1997: 16).

In my terms, the being of essence and persistence in being engages in the *polis* by offering its vulnerability to the *polis'* indifference whilst letting the *polis* take interest in its power of endurance. Simultaneously, it 'abandons' the inessential part of its being, that is, the passivity of being despite itself, to which the *polis,* as an organisation of competing interests, relates with exceptional indifference - as the institution of *Homo Sacer* graphically shows. Further, the 'socialisation' of being in the western *polis* (i.e. the alternance of interest in essence and indifference in pure suffering) to which Agamben refers is of course concomitant with the participation in a *juridical order.* Agamben looks to the obscure Roman institution of *Homo Sacer* to capture this conversion from human animal to juridical *persona*: no less than the 'abandonment', as he terms it, of 'naked' human life to the *polis* through its juridical institutions. Indeed, since Roman times the **social** life of the human animal has become indistinguishable from its *person*alised life, in the juridical sense. In order to become political the human animal must take on the three-fold juridical masks, or *dramatis personae*, of private subject, citizen and member of a social totality. To these three, I argue, correspond the three categories of human rights that the law has progressively come to recognise: civil rights (of property, economic freedom, freedom of expression), political rights (of electing and being elected), social rights (of association, to labour and to strike).

Agamben's views must be re-thought. I have argued that the relationship between 'naked' subjectivity and the *polis* is not exhausted in terms of consciousness and essence, as either one of indifference and solitude or inter-*esse*. There is a further level on which the city and its laws are indeed affected by the 'other side' of subjectivity, as being-for-humanity, but with no recognition and accounting. Can we re-think the presence of the 'naked' human in our society as other than an object of alternating interest and indifference? That we are interested/uninterested in each other's strengths/weaknesses does not of itself show that our society of needs is *not only* a sharing and exchange for the satisfaction of selfish needs *but also* a communion based on disinterestedness. In the words of the Greek writer John Zizioulas, because the notion of 'society' can only convey the interest/indifference that humans may have towards their 'needs', we need to employ the term 'communion of needs' (Zizioulas 1985: 33-34). In such a communion, both the suffering of needs and the responses it demands occur 'for nothing'. In such communion we cry excessively and to no avail for a beloved's death; we remain speechless before the absurdity of our other's excruciating pain. Even our pleasurable love-affairs are intrinsically charitable: we *fall* in love - we give ourselves, put ourselves forth - more than we ever 'are in love' - co-present and committed. In all these circumstances we are not, as it were, 'outside' the circle of interests and commerce that is society. To be sure, there is no intimacy of interests that is not a 'privacy' which already implicates the social. But in proximity one is being social otherwise than through positive/negative implication in another's being and/or having. One is disinterestedly obsessed. One responds for the very absence of meaning of the other's presence and absence, his/her epiphany as a subject of infinite suffering, by offering oneself gratuitously for company and sociality. The other's susceptibility to death and suffering is so absurd one can make no 'commitment' on this basis - albeit you are already for him/her.

Therefore, Agamben's 'implication through exclusion' or 'abandonment' of the human 'naked life' (that is, of its passivity, exposure to risk and mortality) to the indifference of the *polis* must be distinguished from Lévinas' 'disinterested engagement through disengagement', in which there is no implication through negative interest, but only love for alterity. In the disinterestedness and alterity of the one-for-the-other, each being is inessential; it is irreducible to a 'cluster' of common biological/psychological 'needs' (where one is thought to 'be' the needs he/she 'has') or to a subject of essential human rights which come by birth (where one is thought to 'own' the right 'to be'). Being *is* no more than response for the other who, from a position of utter superiority (where 'need' is indistinguishable from 'right'), says 'feed me'. Ethical subjectivity is *not* equal to the needs it is said to 'have' and does not by itself 'own' rights without help; it exists in a communion of needs as a unique 'me' (in the accusative) which answers for its *other's* needs; it only 'has' rights to the extent that another extracts him/her from their circumstances in nature or society, in the process of claiming the compassionate 'right to responsibility' (see my discussion of sterilisation of incompetent women in Chapter 3).

Individualistic rights and generalisable human needs do not, in consequence, allow us to see how heterogeneity requires the being-for-the-other. The *existential heterogeneity* of each human is rather, I submit, to be traced in the *manner* in which beings-*qua*-responsibility are passively (disinterestedly but obsessively) approaching each other. 'Naked life' is lived as traumatic exposure to otherness to which no self-care or collective effort can correspond. The death, illness, hunger and sufferings of all kinds that afflict my other affect *me* in a manner so unique that my cry for help cannot become *logos*. In this sense Lévinas is right that the subjection and expression of absurd, unintelligible human suffering is the 'true knot' of human inter-subjectivity, to the extent of being elevated to a superior ethical principle - 'the only incontestable one - until it governs the spirits and practical disciplines of vast human groupings' (EN: 119).

Therefore to the question 'how does naked life' inhabit the *polis*?' we can no longer answer, as Agamben does: 'by abandoning itself to the interest/indifference of the politico-juridical order'. For the non-essence of 'nakedness' and suffering of being does not simply 'oppose' its interest in persisting in self-containment - it is *superior* to it. Thus, the non-essence of 'nakedness' cannot be fully the object of interest/indifference. In post-phenomenological terms, suffering does not oppose or hinder consciousness - rather, it runs 'counter-clockwise' to it, upsetting it from the inside, coming not 'in opposition to' consciousness and essence but *despite* them. Therefore, nakedness and suffering constitute an irrepressible vulnerability and express an otherwise-than-being which is beyond interest and indifference, when being 'looks up to' its other's 'superior' destitution. Disinterestedness is not an option, but already an undergoing of servitude. Yet the individuated and disinterested manner in which in every instance each social being undergoes its servitude for its uniquely suffering other (in a word, responsibility) cannot by definition concern the *logos* of the *polis*. Agamben is right to point out that the whole edifice of western society relies on each person giving up to the indifference of the *polis* that part of his or her life which cannot be articulated. However, is he right to presume that my self-abandonment automatically does away with my neighbour's disinterested concern?

There exists a manner of expressing one's 'nakedness' which does not betray one's existential heterogeneity. By contrast to *logos,* my inarticulate and inessential cry for help does *not* manifest a perseverance and interest in being to which the *polis* can correspond with selective interest/indifference. The existent's cry for help signifies a subjection to absurd passivity to which *only* the singular neighbour can respond, through substitution, by accounting for this absurdity directly. The subject directly accounts for the absurdity with which its other struggles, in the drama of gratuitous self-giving in which one answers for suffering one has not caused. In this way, the structure in which the *polis* responds with selective interest/indifference to my essence as interest to be gets subverted. In the proximity of being-for-the-absurdly-suffering-other I am disinterested towards my other's essence, but also incapable of showing indifference. I am full of guilt and empty of all essence. I cannot die in the other's place. I cannot cry enough for the absurdity that grasps my other. I am breathless. But 'breathless' does not mean uninspired. I breath the *void* which the other's non-essence leaves, rather than try to fill it with my mourning.

The 'breathless', 'disinterested' subject does not ask questions about its other's needs. My other is more than a cluster of needs. In taking direct responsibility for the absurd nakedness of his/her life I transcend the 'natural' idea of human needs as the infinite pursuit of self-aiming interest. The significance of my other's needs cannot be expressed in the idea of self-perseverance and interest, as it can be in the idea of my infinite responsibility for my other's utter, infinite destitution. The multiplicity of competing human needs must be seen otherwise than as leading 'objectively' to the necessity for a system of law which *delimits* the endless pursuit of self-interest. Such systems recognise these needs as the object of rightful claims by the self-interested individual, while, at the same stroke, they prohibit or ban the 'unmeasured' pursuit of satisfaction: after all, the non-abuse of rights that law grants is an obligation upon the individual. Right and obligation, entrenchment and delimitation of interest, seek to discipline the relations between individuals into a logic of balanced prioritisation of multifarious, additive self-interests. But from the perspective of proximity of the one for the other who is more 'naked' than all his/her needs put together, and to which no self-interest can ever correspond, the requirement for delimitation shifts from the pursuit of self-servitude to that of other-servitude. The function of the law of conventions and contracts is not restricted to regulating the transformation of 'natural' needs to claims of interest.

Law's function is more excessive than necessary, for it generally attempts to impose the sense of measure on the immeasurable and anarchic non-sense which the suffering of one person is for another. The legal delimitation of the unmeasured pursuit of self-interest is not, strictly speaking, delimitation of anything in particular, for such pursuit corresponds to no objective need - need is endless. Rather, what is delimited is the *expression* by the subject of the meaninglessness and absurdity of the very idea of utter self-interest and egoism. So by 'delimiting' what is intrinsically absurd the law gives rise to the belief that the delimited pursuit of self-interest somehow compensates for the absurdity of human vulnerability. Is not the law thus 'banning' or 'exempting' or proscribing indifference towards the expression of meaninglessness by the subject of needs? Is not the law so making it impossible for its subjects to express (and respond to) *useless suffering* ? We hastily call an adult's cry for 'total' help 'childish' and 'irresponsible'. We condemn as hysterical the 'nagging' call for help for what *cannot* be helped. We fear the psychotic pursuit of love. We disregard that these are signs by which the ego shows that its nakedness exceeds its essence as the pursuit of interest. It cannot be stressed enough that in Lévinas such hyperbolic expressions of human suffering are not subsumable under a phenomenology or pathology. To be hysterically, obsessively or psychotically self-concerned or self-destructively resigned to passivity shows the subject, not just as occupying the 'negative side' of its properly objectifiable function or role in the 'social body', but rather as 'otherwise' than a member of a social totality in which only its measured interest and persistence in being are of interest. It is my argument, in conclusion, that the absurdity of human suffering which has no social interest can be ignored but *cannot* be obliterated.

What, then, is the political implication of infinite suffering, exposure and 'nakedness' of each individual being, which cannot be obliterated? If by 'person' we understand *persona*, from the Latin *personare*, meaning the mask worn by an actor through which his voice sounded, then this implication is hard to understand. In the legal theatre of subjectivities, too, subjectivity means solely a social role and function, leaving no space for pure suffering. From a theatrical point of view, the suffering which befalls subjectivity and which abstracts it from its social role and function can have no ethical inter-personal significance. In the theatre of legal subjectivities pure suffering can only go unnoticed or else bring about embarrassment or ridicule. Suddenly, the singer stops singing with a sore throat or the actor unexpectedly falls and cries out: the absurdity of the moment will be appropriated in the embarrassed laughter of the audience or the discomfiture of the unfortunate actor's fellows. Neither of these reactions constitutes an ethical response: how can one *answer for* that absurdity which is not forthcoming into *logos*, and does not get appropriated by what Keenan called the subject of *Vorstellung*, which is 'always' standing up? (see above).

On the other hand, if we follow the Greek for 'person' - *prosopo*, from *prosopsis*: that is, one whose 'face' is always 'turned towards' something or someone - then one *can* be 'turned towards' the 'uselessly suffering' other in a disinterested way. Who cares for the speechless actor's plight? The other in distress is the 'only one that matters' for the one who witnesses it. Who cares for the singer's weak throat or the actor's falling, and their right (more or less) to have their weaknesses respected? These events captivate me in their absurdity, not by their sense. In the 'now' of these events no sound comes through my other's juridical mask. Who/what is behind the mask? Nobody/nothing I may know. Yet, *here I am*, in *prosopsis* with the other, faced with him or her. 'Behind the mask' my other is not simply a cluster of needs to which correspond claims of self-interest. He/she is the constant reminder that *me* responds for the other's passivity. The other's hyperbolic demand for attention, help and care by me includes what he/she cannot possibly have a 'need for', if I understand him/her as a being-for-itself, and what he/she cannot rightfully claim, if I understand him/her as performing a role or function in the multiplicity of self-interested beings which is society. Thus, the *esse*, the other, is the source of my disinterestedness. I am called to *substitute* myself for this inessential but suffering other. By contrast, in the social order that Agamben is describing the essential animal which becomes the abstract juridical persona appears to have resigned its existential heterogeneity. Moreover, in the process of taking up its roles in the politico-juridical theatre and living *as if* a private subject, a citizen and an (additive) member of a social totality, 'the human animal' must abandon not only its 'naked life' but also its absurdly unique, incomparable and dissimilar *manner* of being naked before its uniquely proximate neighbour. In other words, one's nakedness is not only of interest to oneself (as persistent being) and of indifference to the *polis*, it is also a matter of disinterested concern for its neighbour. The socialisation process that Agamben seems to have in mind is therefore too simple. It proceeds directly from 'being' as isolated 'animal' to 'being' as undifferentiated juridical persona, by-passing the impact of proximity between directly affected neighbours.

Lévinas would not be surprised by the fact that the language of law needs to 'abandon' or 'except' that aspect of human life (*zoe*) which cannot be manifested in language, in order to mark its passage to *bios*, the life useful to the *polis*. In language, our delirious 'Saying' *qua* response to the other's absurd life (the life of the animal that does not speak, the life that is of no interest to civilised life) is always ultimately subordinated to the said, to linguistic systems and to ontology, from within which our interested responsibilities to the other as part of Being are accounted for (AE: 6). But if my analysis of the *Bland* case showed anything, it is that ontological discourse is broken only if we shift our focus from the subject's intentional activities-inactivities to its radical passivity. Surprises and adventures are possible because the time of diachrony, of Saying, of delirium and obsession for the neighbour who approaches *before any commitment is in place,* resists its absorption by the simultaneous time of the said, of commitment and synchrony. The self is never active enough either to match the advent of the other in commitment, or to escape it. Something gets *irrevocably lost* and cannot be freely remembered. Being's triumph does not last and one gets older.

The words 'irrevocably lost' must be stressed, for the Lévinasian distinction between 'Saying' and 'said' is not of the dialectic kind. If Lévinas is capable of talking of passive exposure to transcendence, it is because he assumes the human subject as being passively there 'prior' to its ability to playfully separate and associate the Said and the Unsaid. But what is the time of this 'prior'? This 'prior' does not signify antecedence but *diachrony.* By the 'diachronic time of pure passivity' of being for the other (or, the otherwise than being/not being) Lévinas means that 'the temporalisation of time, in the way it signifies being and nothingness, life and death ... must also signify the *beyond being and not being*; it must signify a difference with respect to the couple "being and nothingness".' (AE: 9; my translation). If we note the word 'must' here, the first question to ask would be whether Lévinas is describing two aspects of the *same time* - one being the synchronic and one the diachronic. If yes, what, further, is the meaning of 'must'? Does Lévinas not conflate the diachrony that 'must' be expressed in time with what time 'is'? The answer to the first question is yes. And by diachrony and synchrony Lévinas does refer to the same time, and in that way he remains in the field of essence and metaphysics. He himself says that all time (or rather temporalisation) *is* essence (ibid.). 'Time ... is recuperation of all divergencies, through retention, memory and history. In its temporalisation ... nothing is lost, everything is presented or represented, everything is consigned and lends itself to inscription, or is synthesised, or, as Heidegger would say, assembled, [so that] ... everything is crystallised or hardened into substance' (ibid.). However, time is not merely persistence of essence but also *showing* of essence in the *saying* (ibid.).

This showing remains enigmatic (AE: 10), for *in* the time where the being of substance comes to pass there is also always a 'lapse of time' where the past and origin of acts and speeches are 'irrevocably lost', and there is no way that this origin can be made present by temporalisation. Quite simply, the diachrony of our doing and speaking in time means that we cannot account from within time for the beginning or origin of our actions and speech. Hence time transcends itself: this does not mean that there is recourse to a separate 'kind' of infinite time that runs alongside the time of linear succession of moments in which past and future are gathered in the present, but rather that the quidity of time is 'patience'. It means the *fact* that being in time is not only a matter of active 'assembling' of past and future into the present moment, but also passive exposure and endurance of timelessness. We are subjects of time before being in time, in the sense that we bear passively the 'irrevocable loss' of time's own beginning. In that sense, there is a much deeper past than that of memory and history, a past that we can conceive of without, however, being able to capture its essence through retrospection; and so, we are exposed to a past that cannot be turned into a present, 'a past more ancient than every representable origin, a pre-original and anarchical *passed*' (AE: 9, my translation). My relationship with this past is 'included in the extraordinary and everyday event of my responsibility for the faults and misfortunes of others, in my responsibility that answers for the freedom of another ... [T]he freedom of another could never begin in my freedom, that is, abide in the same present, be contemporary, be representable to me. The responsibility for the other cannot have begun in my commitment, in my decision. The unlimited responsibility in which I find myself both free and hostage come from a 'prior to every memory', an 'ulterior to every accomplishment', from the non-present *par excellence*, the non-original, the anarchical, prior to or beyond essence.' (AE: 10; my translation).

What then - if anything - remains of Lévinas' ethical subject of moral obligation under these circumstances? Following the aforementioned politico-juridical 'abandonment' and 'exclusionary-inclusion' of the other as naked being, the individual's *esse* (persistence-in-being) or *essence* becomes the object of legal (normative) and moral 'indifference' alternating with legal (factual) and political (governmental) 'interest'. The subject's living experience of 'commercial society' (as Lévinas often calls the inter-*esse*) is that of an aggregation of the conflicting (but similar) interests of the various beings. Further, it is consciousness and awareness of the fact that in the above circumstances the being-with-others implies the (supposedly necessary) *alternance* of 'war' and 'commercial' peace; in these circumstances 'peace' is at best the 'synchrony of war' and has no space for obsessive approach, gratuitous charity and love. The institution of law is attractive because it offers a suitable means for such synchrony. In short the rule of law dictates the extent to and the manner in which the interest to be-for-itself is to be exercised between plural beings. It transforms 'war' into 'commercial peace' and establishes an order whereby the various 'essential' human 'needs' are recognised, but, simultaneously, the significance of human suffering is *delimited*. At once acknowledging and reducing the significance of human exposure to suffering, the laws state which human needs can be pursued 'rightfully' and which cannot. The 'reasons' and 'justifications' offered for such selectivity are always absurd, but the consequences are of tremendous importance, since it is out of 'legitimately' acknowledged human needs that politically viable 'rights' emerge: the right to life is thus recognised alongside the right to citizenship, which in turn is linked to procreation. Moreover in such an 'ordered' view of society, the human association is presented as if it were the effect of the individual subject's 'choice': either to take an interest in what the other 'is' or 'has', or to remain indifferent to what the other 'is not'/'has not'. The relationship between the weak and the strong is thought to be based on 'want' and so can be sated with knowledge or in mimetic desire of the 'wanted'. Further, the interest in what the other 'is' and 'has' is underlined by an 'anxiety': the subject of commerce and law must, eventually, be informed also by its other's mortality, that is, by the fact that what 'is' will cease to be, and what 'possesses' will be dispossessed. This *angst* can be 'useful' to the subject in helping it come to terms with what itself 'is not' or 'has not', but it may distract from that which earlier I called 'useless suffering'.

CHAPTER 6

Neighbours

Our community is severed. *Homo Politicus* finds its home in the neighbour's loss (Charles E. Scott in Peperzak ed. 1995: 27).

The other stands in a relationship with the third party, for whom [or for which] I cannot entirely answer ... The other and the third party, my neighbors, contemporaries of one another, put distance between themselves and me and the other, and between the other and the third party (AE: 157; translation modified).

Justice is impossible without the one that renders it finding himself in proximity. His function is not limited to the subsuming of particular cases under a general rule. The judge is not outside the conflict, but is in the midst of proximity. This means that nothing is outside the control of the responsibility of one for the other (AE: 158).

Justice, then, does not arise from an ego, [nor] from a decentering ideal speech situation, [nor] from behind a hypothetical veil, [n]or merely out of community. Rather, it is the normative aspect of exposure to the Other who is neither merely an ego nor a radically situated self. Justice is not the first virtue of social institutions but the ground *and* normative side of sociality that is neither egocentric nor merely communitarian (P. H. Werhane in Peperzak ed. 1995: 65).

I
Obsession with 'informal justice'

In the context of medical law, I have shown in Chapter 3 how the so-called 'justice perspective' is altogether rejected by many in relation to conflicts of values centering on illness-suffering and medical responsibility.[1] But in the last years of the twentieth century the saying that 'lawyers separate' has been heard beyond hospitals. It expresses a much more general anxiety about the effects of the rule of law on community and personal, eponymous relationships. Legal adjudication, even in areas of responsibility with which lawyers are more familiar

---

[1] Remarkably, the claim that the strictures of justice do not suit the ethical character of care was made both from within and without the legal profession: English judges derail medical cases from the path of adversarial litigation, just as the feminist Gillighan declares the unsuitability of procedures aimed at declaring 'right' and 'wrong' for resolving the complex moral problems arising in care.

than they are with medical law, has been obsessively (that is, at least for no
apparent reason) attacked by advocates of Informal Justice through the use of
Dispute Processing or Alternative Dispute Resolution schemes (ADR).[2]
Arguments in favour of ADR were made on the basis of early sociological
conceptualisations of 'formal' law, as well as on anthropological findings.[3] The
main reason for the anthropologists' antipathy towards professionalised court
litigation was that it 'usurps the conflict' by removing it from its immediate
surroundings where the resources for its informal resolution already exist.[4] For the
sociologist, formal law 'transforms' conflict, often unrecognisably to those
involved, into a 'professionalised' legal dispute. Moreover, adversarial court
litigation with its emphasis on rights, liability, guilt and innocence, is thought to
be unable to resolve conflicts in ways which are conducive to the 'restructuring of
damaged bonds between people in on-going, close relationships' (Hogarth 1974,
Becker 1975).[5] In the process, the 'immediacy of dissension is transposed into

---

[2] I use 'Alternative Dispute Resolution' (ADR), or 'Dispute Processing' (DP) as umbrella
terms for a wide range of programmes involving various forms of mediation, arbitration,
conciliation, direct negotiation and reparation that were first set up in the USA, and to a
lesser extent in Britain, in the 1970s.

[3] In his article on 'Formalism' Frederick Schauer sketches out the two main theoretical
streams with regard to formalism. Thus 'formalism' can be conceptualised either 'as the
denial of choice *by* the judge' or as 'the denial of choice *to* the judge' (at 521). Later we
shall see how the 'deconstructionist' approach to legal interpretation by D. Cornell seems
to signify *outwith* the former current. As for ADR which is our concern for the moment, my
understanding of its critique of the 'formalism' of legal adjudication is that it endorses the
latter conception maintaining that '[t]o be formalistic is ... to be enslaved by mere words
on a printed page' (ibid.). I take it that such a position comes as a literal (formal?)
adaptation of Weber's *ideal* description of legal formalism. Weber, indeed, described
formalism as the juridical 'construal' of the 'facts of life in order to make them fit the
abstract propositions of law' in accordance to the maxim that 'nothing can exist in the
realm of law unless it can be 'conceived' by the jurist in conformity with those 'principles'
which are revealed to him by juristic science' (Rheinstein 1954: 304). However already in
the introduction to *Max Weber on Law in Economy and Society* Rheinstein warns us that
Weber's *ideal types* are nominal rather than *real* descriptions of - for that matter - juridical
phenomena. To take 'formalism' non-nominally as the linguistic limitation of the judge's
choice 'conjoins two different elements: mechanical deducibility and the existence of a
closed legal system' of law (ibid. 523: my emphasis).

[4] 'The anthropological and comparative literature performed a dual function. On one hand it
suggested that informalism was essentially a transhistorical phenomenon whose relevance
had mysteriously been lost, while on the other hand it appeared as a relatively recent
development based on the destruction of traditional ideologies and interests. Thus, for
some it acted as a backward-looking reassuring experience, while for others it provides a
futuristic and potentially progressive opinion' (Matthews ed. 1988: 3).

[5] Advocates of informal justice through ADR have never defined properly those
interpersonal 'close' relationships. The relevant literature included no set of criteria or
principles for distinguishing said type of proximity although it appears that 'closeness'

conceptually distant legal categories that render conflict accessible to the courtroom's adversarial rules of procedure. As the trial proceeds, many litigants become further alienated from the process as they bear witness to an emerging 'case', interpretatively constructed by legal counsel and decided upon by the lofty stroke of judicial decision ... The inhospitable atmosphere of what may be called formal, professional calculations of, and practices of justice has something to do with the survival of, and a continued search for, more congenial, informal "alternatives"' (Pavlich 1996: 1).

All in all, in the advocates' discourse, informal justice is rather narrowly associated with 'hospitable' mediation techniques and/or the availability of 'congenial local fora' for the settlement of disputes. Moreover, community-level mediation and negotiation aim respectively at 'conciliation' or 'compromise', rather than proclaiming winners over losers. Furthermore, the argument continues, ADR encourages disputants to work out acceptable settlements voluntarily in cases where the heavy-handed approach of state courts is counter-productive as well as undesirable. It is important that voluntarism features prominently in the relevant discourse. This shows an implicit interest in securing 'lasting' peace, since it is believed that 'agreements that disputants work out themselves are more likely to be followed than those that are imposed by judicial decree' (Pavlich 1996: 56). The intended effect is the 'empowerment' of individual disputants in conjunction with 'strengthening of community ties' (Shonholtz 1988/9). Typically, the resolution of conflicts through the courts' use of what Weber terms 'impersonal' or 'anonymous' law revolves around the juridical concept of rights of property which are individualistic. In consequence, because of the alienation of subject from object that property introduces, the juridical depictions of persons are deemed to be 'too abstract'. In this thesis, one has seen more than one instance, it is claimed (e.g. in the right to refuse medical treatment or the right to reproduce), in which the abstraction of the subject of rights out of its natural/social circumstances has seemed to be too crude, if not absurd.

However, I have argued, from the perspective of rights-as-compassion, that there is no moral problem with the impossibility of justifying the 'ineluctable' violence of human obsession for the other-as-unique. I have argued that a prerequisite for the recognition of the transcendence of human rights is the disinterested and anarchic ('for nothing') approach of the other *as* unique - not yet a commitment *to* an 'abstracted other'. The problem lies, rather, with the absence

---

must include physical contiguity or/and the existence of emotional bonds or micro-economic inter-dependence. Some very crude examples are given. They include couples, family members, neighbours, room mates, landlords and tenants and work colleagues (Pavlich 1996: 57). The closest we come to a fixed requirement is that said relationships should be 'ongoing' irrespective of the eventuality of conflict. But then again it is not clear if this requirement concerns people who want to stay together or have to, or both.

of responsibility regarding the *compassionate* invocation of the other human's rights: then, if reference is made to so-called authoritative, but in reality false reasons and 'truths', the other is objectified. Because false 'truths' and 'authorities' can authorise either good or evil (I have called them, 'principles of absurdity' which appropriate the 'absurdity' of the other's suffering), the activities they guide are only the reverse side of indifference. In law, specifically, judicial irresponsibility gives rise to more than absurd interpretations of the meaning of human rights: it gives rise to a 'principle of absurdity' in relation to how the individuals are legally represented as engaging with one another - as members of a community - in a way which entrenches immorality and indifference. That is, beyond the rights that the subject can claim *for itself*, or those rights which can be claimed for the subject by a judge but only in relation to the subject's self, there *is indifference*. I will be arguing that the substitution in ADR of this kind of subject of rights by the subject of self-interest, does not by itself rescue the subject from the moral 'loneliness' (that is, its being excepted from the ethical order of anarchy that governs the being-for-each-other) in which it is being exiled by law.

Two points must be made. First, the proponents of ADR practice do not distinguish between responsible and irresponsible reference to human rights. For them *all* reference to juridically recognised human rights and obligations must, irrespective of the issue of responsibility, be 'suspended' in relation to conflicts between people in close, on-going relationships. The rights of the other human are replaced in ADR by the notions of 'interests' and/or 'needs'. But even if the 'abstract' juridical rights of my other (i.e. the one that, in ethical terms, *I* mark with an identity of uniqueness) are replaced with 'vital' and 'tangible' counters of subjectivity, the *being-for-each-other* is obscured by egoism. Interests/needs imply their subject to be 'self-embracing' materiality and closure. This subject of interests/needs *is* pure being-for-itself; it is capable of synchrony with other similar subjects albeit only 'spontaneously' and, therefore, 'outside' consciousness and responsibility. In fact, therefore, ADR practices address a 'self-confinable' subject which is incapable of engaging in gratuitous charity and infinite responsibility of the one-for-the-other.

Secondly, it is noteworthy that ADR advocates emphasised the 'time-consuming' nature of state litigation, as against the need of disputants in 'on-going relationships' to have their conflict addressed as a matter of priority. Informal justice is therefore supposed to have a task which is 'more urgent' than the one that the formal kind of justice sets itself; formal law concentrates on the conflict and ignores the even more urgent task of 'ventilating anger' and 'restoring damaged emotional bonds'. This sense of lack of time implies more than a comparison of the real time that passes in court and during out-of-court negotiation/conciliation. It shows that the ontological supposition made by informal justice discourse about the subject, in addition to considering it a 'being-for-itself', includes a *being without time*, or being impatient. In sum, informal justice addresses a being-for-itself which is so occupied by attending to its needs that even in the closest of its relationships it is 'without time' for the other as other. I argue that it is at this point, the point of its supposed 'truth' and 'justification' in relation to a self-obsessed, impatient being, that the ADR discourse becomes mystifying. However, I also submit that beyond its false 'truths' and absurd justifications, in so far as ADR discourse is delirium and registers obsession with a form of justice which is more ancient than a 'recoverable', 'natural' justice, it is an important source of inspiration for an ethical critique of legal representations of proximity. Despite its many theoretical impasses and difficulties, despite its many recursive conceptual loops and the anachronistic accounts which present the self-interested subject of consciousness as if 'original', informalism is also a prophetic discourse, which speaks of a possible future in which, in the words of Lévinas, justice *remains* justice *only* in a society where there is no distinction between those close and those far-off, but in which there also remains the 'impossibility of passing-by the closest' (AE: 158).

ADR proponents took a stance and stated a truth concerning the alterity that obtains between the rigidities of justiciable 'public' associations and the anarchy of the obsessive approach as charity and care. But it has to be recognised that this alterity is 'unsayable' as such. In so far as the site of proximity and justice is *Said* (even when if it is described in this thesis as the human being-for-each other and as constant 'adieu'), it is always universal and public. And in this objective dimension each subject becomes equal to or equivalent to every other. If ADR discourse has a moral significance this is traced in its failures to re-represent the 'proximity' that inspires it. Although 'justice is impossible without the one that renders it finding himself in proximity', the proximity in question is *not* to be identified with the physical/temporal contiguity or the intimate knowledge, or the empathy, between people in 'close/on-going' relationships. Therefore, one may seek a principle whereby even 'formal', 'impersonal' law can nevertheless be said to be sustained by *proximity* between judge and judged, even in the most 'inhospitable' of courtrooms. Further, although 'justice is inseparable' from proximity as the obsessive approach of 'the other' by the *ego*, this approach is not to be mistaken for the ideal placement of the subject of consciousness towards its other, as 'disengaged' through a 'veil of ignorance' (Rawls 1973); nor with the synchrony of dialogue sustained by the desire to communicate (as for instance in Habermas 1987, 1990).

II
The other left in the cold and
brought back into the fold

The informal justice discourse expresses nostalgia for some lost, mythical natural justice whose purpose had been to 'serve' proximity as obsessive approach rather than as reciprocal engagement and social contract. It can even be said of that discourse that, in mourning the loss of the significance of justice as contact with the stranger in 'formal' law, it attempts to fill an even greater alterity or void. In this connection, however, I submit that there is nevertheless an element of counter-intentionality in the ADR proponents' discourse about the 'recoverable past' 'origins' of justice as proximity which is important and intriguing. Philosophically, the fixation of informal justice discourse on peace as commerce of interests/needs and, in particular, with 'on-going' relationships, i.e. with the preservation of achieved contiguity, no matter what injustices this structure helps to maintain, entails a paradox. On the one hand, ADR practices are said to be 'proximity-friendly' because they focus on the subject's everyday, on-going pursuit of self-interest and need-satisfaction. On the other hand, at least in Lévinas' philosophy, the subject of interest (that is the individual as *esse*, *persistence-in-Being* and *essence*) can only be lonely, and also, impatient. But what else is the meaning of solitude if not absence of patience and time? In *Time and the Other* Lévinas assumes that solitude is *not* the result of a deprivation of a previously given relationship with the other or of some presupposition about the other. He shows, first that 'solitude is an absence of time' (ibid. 57). This is because:

> time is not the achievement of an isolated and lone subject, but ... is the very relationship of the subject with the Other. This thesis is in no way sociological. It is not a matter of saying how time is chopped up and parcelled out thanks to the notions we derive from society, how society allows us to make representation of time. It is not a matter of our idea of time but of time itself (TO: 39).

Lévinas also shows that every being is intrinsically alone in that it exists ('facticity' of existence). Indeed, 'One can exchange everything between beings except existing' (ibid. 42).[6] For this reason large human associations based on commerce and reciprocity in the struggle to meet human needs, are governed by rules which maintain an exceptional relationship to individual human existence, since it is *neither* private *nor* public, *neither* pain *nor* satisfaction. In Chapter 5, and more implicitly throughout, I have shown how in the west the simple (biological) existent came to be thought of by the *polis*' laws as that which is 'different but not unique' in perpetual 'exile', untouchable. It remains 'of interest' but only in its inwardness and self-embrace - in which we seek to know how each being 'works on its own' and perseveres in Being. It is also the 'non-object' of

---

[6] 'It is banal to say we never exist in the singular. We are surrounded by beings and things with which we maintain relationships. Through sight, touch, sympathy and cooperative work, we are with others. All these relationships are transitive: I touch an object, I see the other. But I *am* not the other. I am all alone. It is thus the being in me, the fact that I exist, my *existing,* that constitutes the absolutely intransitive element, something without intentionality or relationship. One can exchange everything between beings except existing' (EE: 42).

moral, political and legal *indifference*; it is an individual 'entity' - a member of a totality - but no longer unique Face. Therefore to turn, as 'informal justice' does, towards the existentially lonely being is to turn towards *no-one in particular*. In this aspect, I argue, both 'formal' impersonal adjudication and 'informal' dispute resolution coincide in their ethical consequences. If Lévinas is right, solitude is an *addition* of self to being, as well as an *abstraction* of being from time; it is, in other words, an *excess of being over time*: it is being-for-itself without time for its other. It is in solitary self-attachment that the ego persists in itself, seeking to satisfy its needs and pursue its interests.[7] It is interesting that the soul that impatiently, 'without time', attends to its needs in order to 'settle into itself' is also an ego which associates with others in a 'timeless' way. Hence, the impatient being-for-itself *also* pertains to (in fact is the constituent member of) the order of 'institutional' life, such as the one abstracted in laws which 'do not die' as they are 'timeless'. If am I right in all the above, then, the inter-personal relation as envisaged by proponents of time-efficient and conciliatory ADR does not differ radically from that of the law.

We intuitively understand that even the closest of partners are essentially 'lonely' in so far as their relationship is reduced to inter-*esse* and servicing of each other's needs. Lévinas' thesis on solitude helps us realise the 'loneliness' of the participants in ADR practices who are expected to 'ventilate their anger' and 'deal'. The thesis on solitude applies beyond the physically or linguistically isolated human (the homeless man, say, whose need for a cigarette on a frosty night is not heard by the busy passer-by, or the vegetating patient who cannot speak of needs and wants). His thesis concerns the ontological event of *hypostasis* wherein an existent 'contracts its existing', or, the indissoluble unity between an eponymous existent and the fact of its anonymous existing. It is an event in which a being 'adds itself to the anonymous fact that it exists' and so comes to claim the fact of existing as if an attribute of itself (TO: 43). The subject of informal justice is just such solitary existence in so far as it is presented as ego which is unable to 'depart from itself'. If solitude is tragic it is not so because it is 'deprivation' of a relationship with the other (the sovereign ego is not in any relationship) but because it ends with the ego being 'shut up within the captivity of its identity, because it is matter' (TO: 57). The subject's 'materiality', for Lévinas, consists of this self-returning movement in which the being takes 'pride' and gains 'sovereignty' through imposing its 'materiality' over the facticity of its being-for-the-other (i.e. the affectivity by the other). Solitude, in other words, is non-belonging to the being-for-the-other; solitude is pure being-for-oneself; the ego then becomes 'an enchainment with regard to itself', 'burdened by self-responsibility' - consciousness becomes 'occupation with itself' (TO: 56). Then,

---

[7]It may be, I will shortly argue, that the above 'law' prescribing being to be-for-oneself lies behind the idea of 'conversion to oneself' in Michel Foucault's 'Hermeneutic of the Subject'.

gratuitous charity and aimless obsession for the other - which for Lévinas, and as argued throughout this thesis - constitute the common 'source' of both proximity and justice) are submerged under the finality of responsibility as encumbering *self*-care.

In the light of the above I submit that so-called informal justice practices cannot rectify a situation where the subject feels alienated, alone and 'bare' before formal state law. It is true ADR emerges in response to a situation where formal adjudication, carried out irresponsibly in the sense I have given throughout, appears to have acquired its own *determinism* and places the judge and each of the disputants as fundamentally 'isolated', 'autonomous' but abstract subjects. How is the other 'left in the cold'? The answer lies in all the cases I have previously examined (in particular the case of the man without consciousness, Chapter 1). In the modern legal discourse 'proximity' means either spatial/temporal contiguity or, according to transcendental idealism, it means the ideal 'presence' of another in a conscious representation. As the 'neighbour's coming' is assumed to be ordered by consciousness, law ceases to express the ethical truth that 'commitment is to be defined by approach and not the other way around'. In short, law gives priority to the subject of consciousness by leaving out the subject of suffering and responsibility. When in consequence, consciousness is founded in its own self-positing and self-recuperating movements, in the sameness of law's reflexive movements, alterity and the significance of the one-for-the-other are lost.

This situation, however, is not rectified simply by providing spatio-temporally 'hospitable', non-confrontational, fora for negotiation or mediation which are defined as spaces which exclude the state judge and all he or she stands for. The judge, like any adjudicator, stands for individuated responsibility. The judge also stands for the 'third' in formally representing all the social partners to whom the disputants are responsible; without the presence of a 'third' responsibility cannot be infinite. The judge, *also* stands for the third who nevertheless makes justice possible by finding himself in proximity with the disputants because of the impossibility of passing-by the closest. Therefore, the presence of the disinterested third-as-judge in a relation is necessary as a reminder that justice remains justice only in a society where there is no distinction between those close and those far-off, but in which there also remains the impossibility of passing-by the closest. Hence the figure of the judge as 'outsider' to a conflict symbolises the possibility of beings to be at once close to and distant from, concerned for and disinterested towards each other. In any situation of conflict, I submit, those directly involved need the presence of the disinterested (albeit not 'neutral') 'third' in the middle of their conflict. How else, if not through the intervention of the third, who approaches as a reminder of the infinity of unfinished responsibilities which control the self, can the disputants, in 'close' and 'on-going' relationships, shatter their loneliness and 'get out'? The third-as-judge interrupts the closure of any affair based on interest. The judgement, then, is linked to 'prophecy' and, even, offers *teaching* that being disinterested-for-the-other is possible! But it is a teaching not through 'demonstration' by the judge to the disputants, but in the judge's non-intentional *self-demonstration* and presentation in his or her saying. Is 'informal justice' just according to the above criteria? The answer, I submit, is negative in so far as informal justice presupposes subjectivity to be bound in *self-care* and *self-responsibility* for one's own interests, including emotional stability in on-going close relationships, and the 'needs of the soul'. This situation not only inverts but also 'formalises' the problem with the representation of proximity in 'formal law'. The informal justice discourse (or, for others, 'ideology') 'includes' the other, in the sense that it brings it 'into the fold' of responsibility *as* self-care that which 'formal law' had 'excluded'. It is my argument that in ADR 'ethical subjectivity' as otherwise than being, i.e. as exposure, vulnerability, responsibility and as 'non object' of juridico-political radical irresponsibility and indifference' (as discussed in Chapter 4), *remains* 'in exile'. In informal justice discourse consciousness is founded in its own self-positing and self-recuperating movements almost immediately, as it operates 'blindly' to otherness since it is always consciousness of its own needs.

It is worth reviewing briefly the story of the enunciation and critical reception of the informal justice movement as the attempt to render dispute resolution more compatible with the moral experience of proximity by disputants, and to create a justice model that 'heals' rather than disrupts further human proximity. It is submitted that this attempt was made with haste and spontaneity; as soon as serious reflection had taken place, however, there was a backlash of nihilistic pessimism. Thankfully, it has also been given more sensitive consideration and become the object of constructive scepticism.

III
Between unwarranted optimism and despair

The attitude of informal justice advocates appears to be one of unwarranted optimism. Not having resulted from a well-formulated policy, ADR seemed be a 'practice in search of a theory'. Lacking a properly formulated theory, informal justice was launched as 'an idea whose time had come' (R. Matthews ed. 1988: editor's intro. 2). In so far as some justifications for informalism *were* forthcoming, these were characterised by 'recursive conceptual loops' (Pavlich 1996: 57). The claim that informal justice was an 'independent alternative' to the state's justice system has not been sustained. In this regard, despite the great variety of their formulations, critics have shared a view of informal justice as a residual feature of 'state justice', at a time when the state is expanding and intensifying its control over individuals. The calculations that license ADR practices are best understood as 'harmony ideology' and the 'ADR explosion' is said to have serious implications in diverting attention from the necessity for legal reform (Nader 1988). Moreover, this expansion is said to be 'insidious through a process that, on the surface, appears to be a process of retraction' (Santos 1982: 262). In advocating a shift away from confrontation and litigation to 'harmonious' forms of dispute settlement, the ideology equates 'peace' with 'consensus' in relation to the status quo of actively functioning local communities and close relationships. This is an extremely conservative ideology which has the effect of neutralising the potential of inter-personal conflict to act as catalyst for redressing the subordination of disadvantaged members of community and partners in relationships. Similarly, Abel talks of reducing the 'potential for social disruption' (Abel 1982: 288). Another commentator argues that there is 'considerable evidence that members of communities [actually] *prefer* the authoritative decisions of the courtroom above informally reached settlements because the former can potentially redress power imbalances between litigants' (Tomasic 1982: 229-230; my emphasis). By focusing on individuals in conflict, the informal justice calculations help to individualise disputes that may have structural roots by offering somewhat superficial resolutions (Abel 1982: 286). As an example we can think of spousal abuse; as L. Lerman observes, women enter ADR sessions carrying the burden of 'structurally based oppression' that is unlikely to be addressed by ADR sessions (Lerman 1984).

M. Galanter (1981) and S. Silbey and A. Sarat (1989) focused more on the concepts that ADR advocates employed, in order to demonstrate the interdependence of juridical, abstract and individualistic 'rights' and their informal 'alternative', i.e. 'interests' and 'needs'. In this connection, Silbey and Sarat found a high degree of theoretical naiveté in the arguments in favour of ADR, and even in conclusion charged the sociologists who argue against formal litigation with acting out of professional interest (in wishing to extend their competence into traditionally legal domain)! Galanter focused on how informalism misleadingly 'naturalises' the experience of grievance and conflict before doing the same with their resolution in intimate 'local fora'. He talks of a vertical 'continuum' or 'vast and uneven pyramid' where conceptions of disputes emerge gradually out of 'injurious' experiences only by means of dependence on social/legal categories which give rise to dispute and justice speculations alike (Galanter 1981: 12). The perception of grievances requires cognitive resources, Galanter writes (ibid. 14), and what people perceive as 'injurious depends on current and ever-changing estimations' (ibid. 13) of what enhances or impairs health, happiness, reputation etc. These estimations are qualitatively indistinguishable from those employed by formal law and state courts. Those experiences that are not cognitively constituted as 'deserved punishment' or as the result of assumed risk or fickle fate, are instead constituted as 'violations of some rights or entitlement' (ibid.). Moreover, Galanter argues, the calculations of justice in terms of interests and needs in negotiation or mediation processes do not differ radically from formal adjudication on the basis of rights. Simply partaking in a society of state law and courts endows people's private negotiations and mediations with a 'bargaining' modality akin to litigation. Conciliation and compromise are reached on the basis of interests/needs only as an alternative 'bargaining counter' to rights.[8] All in all, '[A]djudication provides a background of norms and procedures against which negotiation and regulation in both private and government settings takes place' (Galanter 1981: 32). More importantly, just as in formal adjudication the parties are abstracted as if entities comprised of rights and obligations, informal bargaining processes endow the parties with token interests/needs through which they are expected to understand themselves and eachother (ibid. 33).

Silbey and Sarat's jurisprudential perspective allows them to focus on how ADR advocates had naturalised the concept of dispute and inter-subjective peace. The disputants' needs/interests were taken *as if* neutral referents. Supposedly, people can continue to 'be themselves' if given the chance to articulate the truth about their relationship and their conflict in such 'neutral' terms. For Weber formal law operates as an impersonal, anonymous structure of legal procedures and general legal prescriptions whose rationale allows us to pass from fragmented perceptions and representations of power-contingent and essentially irrational elements of inter-subjective associations to 'pure', 'neutral' concepts. This 'legitimating function' of formal law appears to Silbey and Sarat to be equally performed by informal justice practices. In this connection, they note how the notions of subjective interests and needs on which ADR relied 'take on a meaning only as theoretical counterweights to rights', or as 'alternative basis for claims of rights' (Silbey and Sarat 1989: 498). The idiom of formal justice had hitherto been deployed in terms of rights which may 'seem to constitute an alienating individualism', yet they 'create a recognisable way to understand social life, that is what constitutes "we", rather than solely "me" ' (ibid. 490). But, 'there is a way in which rights make possible the kind of community, interaction and connection

---

[8]'Negotiation' and 'compromise' are exposed as *traditional* forms of dispute resolution. Seventy per cent of those who experienced 'middle range' grievances made claims for redress, that is, they spoke directly to the injurer in order to settle the issue before recourse to a third person or authority. Of those claims that end up as disputes 'a large portion ... are resolved by negotiation between the parties'. Almost half of the disputes in the Miller and Silbey and Sarat survey ended in 'agreement after difficulty' which at least Galanter takes as indicating the occurrence of negotiation. In sum, 'Negotiation ranges from that which is indistinguishable from the everyday adjustments that constitute the relationship to that which is bracketed as a disruption or emergency' (Galanter 1981: 16-17). Negotiated settlement is an integral part of dispute resolution in all embedded fora which 'process a tremendous number of disputes' (ibid. 17) and it even takes place 'in the anteroom of the adjudicative institution' (ibid. 27): i.e. in the instance of 'plea bargaining' in American law. 'Plea bargaining', as described by Galanter, resembles substantially the 'alternatively' proposed mediated settlement or the negotiated compromise respectively, according to the role of the judge in the plea who 'may be passive, merely ratifying deals arranged by the parties; (or) ... may actively participate in plea discussions; or ... may play a dominant role' (ibid.).

sought in the [informalists'] discourse of needs/interests at the very moment that they seem to encapsulate individuality, separateness and difference' (ibid.). All in all, rights are 'transformed, and in some ways domesticated in the face of the discourses of needs and interests', and the subject of interests 'replicates the contradiction between self and other which plagues the rights conception' (ibid.497).

For supporters of informal justice the significance of the neighbour is reduced to one of spatial/temporal contiguity, and his or her presence is identified with the conscious presentation of interests/needs to which corresponds the 'pastor's' care and protection through advice and help. In reverse, for the 'social-constructionist' critics of 'informal justice' the significance of the neighbour as pastor is to be derived entirely from social history. But in either, I argue, no case is made against the contention that:

> the neighbour's proximity does not originate in any intentional synthesis.. [Moreover] He or she does not occur first as poor or powerful or deprived or victim. or attractive or curly-headed ... His or her proximal but unpresent touch assesses and persecutes consciousness ... An act of consciousness is delayed in its self-enactment before the neighbour who, being without a who or consciousness, is timelessly before the act of consciousness that unavoidably bestows time and presence on the neighbour. The neighbour is before the before, unlost before being lost, utterly unpolitical before its political beginning and consciousness. The neighbour renders us speechless in giving us to speech ... denies consciousness the identity of its self-enactment in giving its identity. It breaks the truth of consciousness, its self-disclosure (C. E. Scott in Peperzak ed. 1995: 27).

Whilst it is reconfirmed that:

> Foundering in its struggle for recuperation, consciousness, which is always political, finds itself without the authority necessary to found an order for the neighbour and *loses the neighbour in recognising the neighbour*. Whatever consciousness does regarding the neighbour, it contaminates by ordering the neighbour's coming: by orders of respect and benevolence, by orders of generosity, greeting, concern, protection and nurturance. [However] No politics will reinstate the neighbour's touch. We are lost before we began. Our community is severed. *Homo Politicus* finds its home in the neighbour's loss (ibid.).

IV
'Seeking Ego without adversity'

How would Lévinas view the 'essentialist' aspect of ADR and how view its critics' 'social-constructionist' perspective? First of all, Lévinas is neither an essentialist nor a 'social-constructionist'. The self, for him, is neither essence prior to socialisation nor, however, is it an outcome of socialisation. Nor can the self be reduced to an ideal presence in a discourse. From this point of view it is not so important to accuse the proponents of informal justice of helping to maintain the social status quo, with all its injustices, through reiterating an essentialist view of the human subject and denying that the subject is 'radically situated'. It is more interesting to explain how the aspiration for a justice which 'heals' proximity becomes *entangled* with what Adrian Peperzak has called 'egology' i.e. the focus on the subject of self-interest as the centre of the being and as source of philosophy, ethics and moral judgements (Peperzak 1993: 46).[9] The story, from the enunciation of the aspiration for 'community justice', through to its dismissal as extending state control, revolves around the problem of individuation and universality. The latter, in turn, is played in the contemporary debates as a philosophical need to discern the primacy of either one of the two components of a dilemma between morality/justice, responsibility/rights, or community/individual. The problem of 'egoism', one of the most difficult notions in ethics, is, however, tackled by Lévinas precisely because he does not work his way from a starting point such as the ego, the individual or the cogito. '[T]he confrontation with the other is both irreducible and linguistic, as exposure which is both normative and empirical' (AE: 48). Exposure to the other is both constitutive of human experience *and* its ground. Lévinas writes that 'at least in the first instance; Being is exteriority' (TaI: 290).[10] Nevertheless, 'egology' continues to be a problem and it is important to remind ourselves of the degree to which it has:

> influenced social philosophy as well philosophies [such as those of John Rawls and Jürgen Habermas]. A central issue in the debate, simply put, is this: what is the relationship between the individual and the community? No one disputes the fact that one is born within and initially influenced by one's community, culture, and society. But is the self merely a product of and determined by community, 'radically situated' such that what it does is merely an outcome of complex interrelationships in which it is continually engaged? If so, it is not easy to explain how it is that we are self-reflective, self-critical, creative makers of history, and authors of change ... If [by contrast] the self develops or can exert itself in a form of disengagement from community, does it become so radically different as to become merely a Sartrian *pour-soi* ? If so, individuals, as disembodied selves, cannot make choices that are more than spontaneous acts rather than rational decisions based on knowledge, context and past experience. It is not merely Sartre who holds this view. For example, John Rawls argues that rational persons behind a hypothetical

---

[9] For more, see my Introduction, n. 7.

[10] Moreover, Lévinas does not begin with community language or convention 'as Wittgenstein does ... Nor does he start from a metaethical intuitive foundation such as Rawls's statement that 'justice is the first virtue of social institutions'. Rather Lévinas begins with 'face to face', the confrontation with the Other' (OB: 18-19). This confrontation is both descriptive and normative, and who one is and how justice is defined become realised only in this confrontation (Werhane in Peperzak ed. 1995: 63).

'veil of ignorance' where they are 'disembodied' from their history, race, ethnic origin, religion, gender, and social class, can develop principles of justice that apply to real people embedded in social situations. But can a mere subject self actually engage in thinking about such concrete notions as theories of justice? Underlying Rawls' project is the presupposition that society does not contribute to selfhood, although a collection of selves creates society. But then, how does community develop at all from this collection of radically disembodied subjects? (Werhane in Peperzak ed. 1995: 60-61).

It is my argument that, following Lévinas', one can go beyond the posing of such dilemmas. For instance, from a non-egological point of view one can be sympathetic to both informalists and their critics, but *not* agree with their egological premises. The 'other' whom formal law allegedly ignores and which informal justice aims to serving, is neither an object of social production nor a 'disembodied' subject which, like a vegetating patient or Orestes-in-exile or a positivist judge, operates as pure abstraction. Patricia Werhane is absolutely right that John Rawls' *A Theory of Justice* presupposes such an abstract subject of justice in his hypothesis of a 'veil of ignorance'.[11] Yet, to the question 'can a mere subject self actually engage in thinking about such concrete notions as theories of justice?' (Werhane in Peperzak ed. 1995: 60) Lévinas would give a negative answer. If, as I hold, 'obsession', 'charity' and judgment are all inseparably connected, the presupposition of a 'veil of ignorance' by Rawls is *redundant*, whilst Habermas' 'ideal speech situation' seems excessive. Why should passive, disinterested engagement through disengagement with the other be idealised, and be thought of as the active indifference, and/or the charming modesty of Rawls' subject which, in all virility, can simply 'put on' a veil of ignorance? Why convert being's passive exposure to its other into a (necessarily) circular ontological presupposition about the subject of consciousness? Behind the veil of ignorance the subject is 'disembodied', that is, abstracted from its community, but remains capable of developing principles of justice which apply to real people in real situations; but this is the position of the sober theorist who overlooks humanity from a higher ground and therefore is not emotionally immersed in it.

Why must we assume a subject 'beyond adversity'? Why must we assume that the subject desires to and can and must 'communicate'? Is this not the position of

---

[11]'Jürgen Habermas['s response] to Rawls' problem with the notion of 'progressively 'decentred understanding' of the world through which one aims at a more universal moral discourse from an 'ideal speech situation'. The process of decentering develops from one's initial pre-conventional stage of self-interest and individuation that originates from socialisation. This view ... comes closer to Lévinas's perspective, yet it does not yet fully resolve the dichotomy between the self and community ... [I]t is not clear that either Habermas or Rawls establishes Lévinas's argument that the essence of morality (and thus of justice as well) is 'first philosophy'. [This view offers] ... an intuitive assumption not a ground' (Werhane P.H.1995 in Peperzak ed. 1995: 61).

Keenan's 'subject of *Vorstellung*' which, it is assumed, 'must be' and, for that matter, be-*for*-itself', and 'speak of' or otherwise communicate its suffering, mostly in terms of 'vital rights', or alternatively 'rightful interests', and which brings shame to those who remain speechless before the 'scandal' of human suffering and are often 'moved' obsessively? Are we not, due to death and the impossibility of dying in each-other's place, responsible even *for the non-response* of the dead and for the *non-sense* of suffering? Jürgen Habermas' 'ideal speech' describes perfectly, though obviously for different purposes, the position of such talkative and social if un-emotional being. His situation of the subject within an 'ideal speech situation' does not yet express the pre-originary ethical position of the subject of responsibility and language *as* the subject of *exposure* and of *adversity*. I have shown in relation to the doctor-patient relationship that the definitive event of proximity-as-responsibility is neither contained in what is said between them about suffering nor is it equal to the (finite) human desire to communicate. That event is, rather, infinite and obsessive compassion for the non-sense and evil of human suffering. Going back to the issues with informal justice I disagree that 'close' relationships need be excepted from legal adjudication *in so far as* the latter constitutes a proper forum for the 'confrontation with the Other'; yet I have shown in my discussions of medical law that it is possible that the courtroom ceases to offer such a forum of confrontation between self and other, mainly because of the restriction of the idea of responsibility beyond intentional harm and negligence *for* the otherwise-than-being/non-being. Disinterested approach is thus perversely replaced by the alternation of calculated silences and utterances about the 'transcendental' rights of the other. Supposedly, the judge 'must' recognise rights, rather than admit that he/she chooses to impute to the other such rights in order to exercise his/her own - and perhaps sole - right: 'the right to responsibility'. According to the premises of this thesis, however, in so far as it is denied that the rights of my other flow from my 'right to responsibility', we face, not transcendental identity (as the law would have us believe) but rather, *transcendental loss of identity* (see Chapter 5 on the subjectivity-in-exile). This is how indifference and interest for what the other is/is not and has/has not can usurp the anarchy of judicial individuated responsibility. But this is no reason to replace courts with local fora, and judgement with compromise or conciliation.

The other-in-exile, whose absurd essence (persistence in being for itself) is appropriated by discourses which claim the 'transcendence' of human rights and of the laws that sanction them, gives rise, as essence, to an 'interested' commitment by the western juridico-political order. At the same time he or she is an object of 'indifference' and repudiation of his or her being-beyond-essence. This otherwise-than-oneself must, so to speak, be 'brought in from the cold' - but not 'back into the fold'. Ethics demand more than a conscious act of inclusion of the other by me (which is also, necessarily, a suspension of what in the other cannot be the object of my intentionality). Ethics demand of me, I am afraid, a

responsibility to each other *qua* neighbour and already *my* neighbour, even prior
to our introduction and even before his or her moved into the neighbourhood.
When the courtroom (but equally, the forum of ADR) is 'cleansed' from
responsibility as excessive emotion for the non-essential other as neighbour 'in the
unknown' (see Chapters 1, 2 and 3) it appears a mere theatre of abstractly
autonomous *dramatis personae*: Anthony Bland, Ms Yetter, Ms Northern, Ms
Sidaway, B ... The performance becomes tediously repetitive: it perverts the
responsibility of the subject and, what is more, it makes the work of justice seem
indifferent to humanity *qua* approach of the one for the other; by contrast, it
shows that justice becomes excessively interested in the human ego. *Perhaps*,
then, and for this we must give it the benefit of the doubt, the aspiration of the
'informal justice movement' proponents incorporated a misplaced moral concern
with the failure of the modern western state legal system to acknowledge that
proximity 'shatters' the loneliness of the individual as additive member of the
inter-*esse* of ideas and needs. If the modern 'formal' adjudicator pretends to
occupy a position outside the conflict before him or her, and not outside the
disputants' proximity, a position from which he or she can focus more on
proclaiming winners or losers, this, then, is *not* doing justice. But also, it must be
stressed against the informalists that the solution does not lie in expelling
proximity from the order of justice, as the isolationist survival-as-closure of
socially disconnected subjects of interests in 'close', 'on-going' relationships
suggests.

V
Of pastors converting the being-for-the-other
into a 'collective good'

A non-nihilistic yet sceptical view of informalism is also available. Thus, Peter
Fitzpatrick has argued that 'informal justice' is *neither* an autonomous domain
where conflicts and resolutions occur 'naturally' and individuals remain
'themselves', *nor* is it a 'mere' 'residuum of state power' (1988, 1991, 1993).[12] To
be sure, the self-presentation of the informal justice movement as offering an
'alternative' to the order of state justice is described in terms of 'mythological
homologies' between the two. Despite claims to be alternatives and even in
opposition to one another, the discourses of both formal and informal justice
appeal to central mythical figures. These include the reference to a pre-legal
'natural pre-existing' community and sociality which the law-bound society of
political contract has supposedly come to supersede, and which informalism
recovers or revives. The 'suppression' and the 'revival' occur by means of

---

[12]In fact, he analyses this divide by reflecting on two linked forms of power in modern
societies (Fitzpatrick 1988).

reference to an equally mythical 'autonomous, self-actualising individual' which understands its own and its others' actions through, respectively, rights and interests/needs.[13] More importantly for the purposes of this section, Fitzpatrick argued that informal justice is part of a developing trend towards 'decentralised' modes of exercising power in liberal democratic states. He points to the receding significance of hierarchical, centralised models of power that purported to emanate from a central force. ADR is presented as a 'disciplinary' form of power which operates in local, micro contexts of sociality structuring the traditionally 'private' social spheres where individuals act intimately. Informalism is described as helping to preserve the 'synoptic' hegemony of the law over 'on-going' micro-alliances and struggles. The allegedly 'law-less' natural community and the 'close', 'on-going' relationships of which informalists speak, thus become spaces in which the individual subjects, far from being natural, are continually moulded by techniques of disciplinary power.

In short, informal justice enunciates a particular mode of what Michel Foucault called the 'governance' of collectivities that is different from the law-sovereignty model of power. Accordingly, the modern individual's most personal judgements about its *preservation* involve and are informed by public 'knowledges' and 'discourses'.[14] For Foucault the rise of modern societies is distinguished by the emergence of 'disciplinary knowledges' whose 'object' is the biological individual, i.e. the subject of exposure to natural plagues. This individual, who could very well be Levinas' *vivant*, or Agamben's *naked life*, is thus placed as a singular entity of and as organically connected to a collective 'population'. The emergence of these technologies is most noticeable in numerous institutionalised discourses including those of psychiatry and medicine (Foucault 1979: 14); and even that of informal justice (Foucault 1988: 168). According to this model, the object of governance is comprised of 'singular', albeit also 'additive' or interchangeable existents or entities whose 'well-being' is equated to their 'collective' strength. Under such conditions the significance of the public/private dichotomy is changed. The notion of governance expands the idea of state power well beyond the state's formal apparatus, incorporating the

---

[13]As such, the operations of both formal and informal justice constitute complementary or co-extensive attempts to regulate social action. In this connection it is interesting to recall the myth of Orestes in Aeschylus' play on the 'first legal trial'. As we saw there, 'formal' law never quite supersedes its 'natural' (consuetudinary) or religious predecessors; instead, it incorporates their force. The belief in the possibility of supersession overlooks the mythical dimension of the pre-origins of justice where these are cast in the modality of hint and allusion to a quite different way of encountering the other.

[14]"What do we need in order to keep our control in the face of the events that take place? We need 'discourses': *logoi*, understood as true discourses. Lucretius speaks of the *veridica dicta* that enable us to thwart our fears and not allow ourselves to be disheartened by what we believe to be misfortunes ... discourses enable us to face reality' (Michel Foucault, 'The Hermeneutic of the Subject' in Rabinow ed. 1994: 99).

dissemination of knowledges aimed at 'disciplining' individuals in their most intimate relation to themselves and to their proximates. Peter Fitzpatrick, however, also argues that formal and informal justice discourses are not merely interdependent but also 'specifically resistant' (Fitzpatrick 1993). Such micro-contexts or inter-subjective spaces as informalism sought to colonise are described by Fitzpatrick as more than sites where disciplinary powers integral to the continued existence of the liberal state and its legality are exercised; informal justice is only partially constituted by the legal field; it remains 'un-embedded' and a possible basis from which to resist the hegemony of formal legality.

These views are adopted and further elaborated by G. C. Pavlich (1996). Pavlich revisits the whole issue of the introduction of informal justice procedures from a 'post-modern perspective' and points to how, in 'secular worlds under postmodern conditions', the 'aim of purchasing justice' no longer coincides with securing the proclamation of *lex eterna* or eternal and singular justice (ibid. 1). It is the main feature of post-modern or 'critical' scholarship engaging in legal thought that it suspends all those 'meta-narratives' which traditionally associate the workings of the law with the promise of equal treatment to all those who come before it.[15] Alluding too to Foucault's ethics,[16] Pavlich claims that although informalism must be understood in its disciplinary function as a historically modern phenomenon, it nevertheless also contains an 'ethos' which can be put to 'emancipatory' use.[17] Indeed, Michel Foucault desired the 'permanent reactivation

---

[15]Pavlich cites Lyotard and Thebaud (1985), Derrida (1992) and White (1987/8), all of whom are scholars intent on replacing this traditional promise that law makes to disputants with an ethical and political duty to rectify their circumstances 'in the here and the now'. Moreover, these are writers who reject Rousseauist views on equality as well as the 'phonocentric' belief which assumes that it is possible for individual subjects to resolve their differences in a manner that 'transcends' their structural inequalities provided they operate in circumstances of free speech (e.g. negotiation and mediation in ADR). For Lyotard the right to a fair hearing, for instance, does not do away with subordination: the defendant must 'speak in the language of his or her oppressors'. In this theoretical climate Pavlich explains the phenomenon of informal justice in terms of a disenchantment with the 'liberal promise of equality before the law [which] today rings as little more than a formal, hollow abstraction, largely favouring those with the means to play the game' (ibid.). Informalism emerges in the contradiction between this *lex eterna*, or law as eternal justice, and the operations of *lex temporalis* or law in its everyday operations that passes for justice.

[16]For an introduction to Foucault's approach to responsibility and ethics see Rabinow ed. 1997.

[17]In this regard Pavlich points out that Foucault's thesis recognises:

'no absolute point to ground critique or the emergence of a better society for the future, although he does provide the rudiments of a non-absolute ethical theory in his later texts ... For him, politics involves an ongoing critique of the present limits of our society. We must continuously ask ourselves, 'How can we exist as rational beings, fortunately committed to

of an attitude - that is, of a philosophical ethics that could be described as a permanent critique of our historical era' (Foucault 1984: 42). This critical attitude 'entails an unending diagnosis of the "dangers" that accrue from present limits in social contexts ... [A] series of critiques on an ongoing basis, seeking out the perils imminent in power relations' (ibid.).[18] In this connection Pavlich argues that:

> The practical attempt ... to develop an alternative politics of dispute resolution, would involve no less than the radical *disarticulation of the pastoral and sovereignty-law models*, especially at those moments where their conjunction fortifies (complements) professional calculations of the just. The calculation of a popular, community justice would thus involve - to return to Derrida for the moment - an experience of the impossible, of the silences beyond current enunciations licensed by the governmental state ... Such is the monumental scale of reconstitution involved ... No doubt the uncoupling of the political rationalities requires a form of resistance that is unlikely to be completed by staying within, and is made considerably more difficult by the subtle techniques of, regulatory forms under post-modern conditions. Even so, beginning such a task implies at least two forms of knowledge. First, it requires us to conceptualise resistance in the realm of community justice; because the exercise of power here is *not always visible*, conceptions of resistance should be sufficiently assiduous to take account of the seemingly invisible. Secondly, to avoid the implicit political apathy of the early critics [of informal justice], it is important to ask the question: what strategically can be done? The emphasis here is on the word 'can', to emphasise the speculative nature of my remarks here (Pavlich 1996: 145-146).

Specifically, Pavlich is alluding to the possibility of *subverting* what Foucault called the 'pastoral model of power' (Foucault 1981), in the context of ADR and in relation to the role of the 'community mediator' who focuses on the disputants' needs and interests. As Pavlich says, 'the production of disciplinary knowledges [through the exercise of 'pastoral' power] serves to define *both* singular *and* collective regulatory objects that facilitate the efficient administration to

---

practising a rationality that is unfortunately crisscrossed by intrinsic dangers?' (Pavlich 1996: 102).

[18]From this perspective, Pavlich asserts the proper critique of informal justice requires that all modern 'meta-narratives' about a singular and universally premised 'Justice' must be abandoned. Instead one must develop contextually relevant means of 'assessing the perils and merits' of informalism in relation to the 'radically situated' subject since 'for those who must endure the torment of ongoing conflict, whose resolution is only ever partial and unsatisfactory, there is little need to speak of justice in any abstract sense' (ibid.). In short Pavlich abandons the possibility of a transcendental critique of informalism and adopts a *historically specific* immanent critique. In this connection his emphasis is on what 'must be done' in order to retain ADR practices without 'fortif[ying] professional calculations of the just' (ibid.).

strengthen the state' (Pavlich 1996: 109; my emphasis). The mediator *qua* modern 'pastor' 'attends to the different emotional and other needs, interests and perceptions of each congregant *for the purpose* of reconciling singular regulatory beings with the collective totality' (ibid. 113; my emphasis). All in all:

> If post-modern conditions thrive on haphazard and unlicensed uses of pastiche in architectural design, artistic creations, social events and so on, one could then also point to the *(re-)use* of political models from *erstwhile* patterns of association. Traces of a pastoral model of power ... are related to the Hebraic image of a single God with kings as mortal deputies. Such traces become more definable presences in early Christian societies that organise associative patterns around the church and pass local leadership to pastors. Unlike magistrates, these pastors are enjoined to take an *active interest* in the individual lives of all congregants much as shepherds ... are required to take care of a flock. Pastoral leadership, that is, requires detailed knowledge of each individual life, so that it can be conditioned and nurtured in various ways, thereby securing the well-being of all within the group. Like a shepherd, the pastor must attend to the needs of the entire 'flock' by counselling each seeker, calming the disquieted, resolving conflicts between antagonists, admonishing the wayward, caring for the sick, helping the poor and so on. As such, pastoral leadership 'involves a power which individualises by attributing, in an essential paradox, as much value to a single lamb as to an entire flock (Pavlich 1996: 107; my emphasis).

In the above quotation I have highlighted the word 're-use'. But if Giorgio Agamben (see Chapter 5) is right in claiming that the modern constitution of biopolitics around the biological individual begins already with the establishment of the classical Greek politico-juridical order which 'excludes through including' the individual's 'naked life', then the reference to the 'pastoral' model of power becomes more complex than the one Pavlich suggests with the word '(re-)use'. My first point, in this connection, is that what Pavlich calls 'erstwhile' forms of association and the pastoral model of politics (centring on the individual's needs) cannot simply be 're-used' in post-modernity, as Pavlich suggests, because *they were never out of use*. They must have always remained of use to the law-sovereignty model, albeit as that which the sovereignty model excluded as 'exceptional' and fleeting - say in the clemency of the king or the modern sentencing judge who, in granting pardon or considering mitigation, engages in an 'economy' of affectivity toward human suffering he encounters, alternating between taking an interest in the other's limited being-for-itself and displaying an indifference to the other as infinitely vulnerable. It is therefore more interesting to look at the late modern phenomenon of 'reviving' informal justice, not as a critical point in historical recurrence where the past becomes actual once again, but as the effect of denying the transcendence that *de-measures, obsesses* and *upsets* the institutionalised (legally fixed) economy of compassion and discipline of the being-for-each-other *from the inside.*

Secondly, if it is true that the original political act is one of 'interest in' being's solitary existence and timelessness (essence and perseverance in being), which is at once an indifference and irresponsibility towards otherwise-than-essence, then the 'pastoral' model of informal justice discourse also enunciates a politics in which the 'pastor' attends to the other's sufferings, not gratuitously and 'for nothing', but for the purpose of 'reconciling the other as individual with a totality'. In this regard 'pastoral' care exemplifies the perverse conversion of the ethical command to show disinterested compassion for one another's sufferings into the rule of *selective interest* - the spirit of which is captured by the sophist Epictetus.[19] Finally, when Pavlich analyses community mediation by using the role of 'pastor', he implies that the subject of leadership and initiative, responsibility and care attends to the neighbour's individual interests and needs 'in order to' sustain coherence in the social group; in so doing he is giving us a concrete example of the subject who is 'free' (in ethical terms) and also 'obliged' (in terms of consciousness) to 'depart from itself' for the sake of attending to its others; but, whose care is also, inevitably, a *return to itself*. From the point of view of subjectivity as consciousness this is an ability and 'freedom', whereas from an ethical perspective, by contrast, 'self-return' is not a sign of freedom but of slavery to fate and inevitability.

Who can attend to its other's needs without becoming 'pastoral'? Let me review, first, what the 'pastor' *is*. In 'The Hermeneutic of the Subject' Michel Foucault traces the pastoral role, through its many transformations, back to the Ancient Greek practice of *epimeleia heautou* ('care for the self'; in Latin: *cura sui*), and to Socrates who exemplifies 'the man who takes care that his fellow citizens take care of themselves' (Rabinow ed. 1994: 93). At this point, it is worth considering that Socrates' last *political* act was that of his *resignation* to his death sentence. The principle that one needs to 'attend to oneself' corresponds to and supplements the principle 'know yourself'. In other words Socrates 'gives over' his existence to the *polis* and does so as a form of 'taking care of his soul'; Socrates also 'takes care' that his fellow citizens learn the same lesson. However, it is also worth remembering that, as I pointed out in Chapter 1, Socrates was surrounded not only by his students who were being taught a 'sober lesson', but also by Apollodorus and the women who cried more than one ought, without measure; as if humanity were not subject to measure and there is an excess to politics in death.

Foucault also pointed out how pastorship becomes specifically Christian through orthodox theology which turned the principle of care of the self into a 'constant practice' so that '[A]ttending to oneself is not just a momentary preparation for living; it is a *form* of living one should be, for oneself and throughout one's existence, one's own object' (Foucault in Rabinow 1997: 96). It is linked to the idea

---

[19]See the opening page of my Chapter 5 (top).

of conversion to oneself [*ad se convertere*], the idea of an existential impulse by which one turns in upon oneself [*eis heauton epistrophein*]. Of course the theme of *epistrophe* is typically Platonic. [But whereas Platonic self-return] is an impulse by which the soul turns to itself and by which the gaze is drawn 'aloft'. [T]he turning that [concerns us here is] ... a kind of turning in place; it has no other end than to settle into oneself, to 'take up residence in oneself' and to remain there (ibid.).

We know, then, that the 'pastor' is the subject and teacher of practices directed to self-coincidence through 'care of the self' as well as a fundamental component of communities based on interest, i.e. of societies in which the needs of the individual are of interest in so far as addressing them adds to the 'collective' well-being of the community in which this individual belongs as additive 'member'. It is my argument that the pastor's 'Achilles' heel', in having his function subverted, is that the 'pastor' is *also* the one whose compassion must be de-*limited* beforehand by law in such way as to not extend beyond the individual's 'needs'; pastoral care, I argue, is not entitled to address the other's infinite destitution and absurd suffering. The 'pastor' has a role only in a community of beings who are 'settled' and 'at home' with one-another, without rupture in their truth, without revelation, without obsession, surprise, anarchy, and without responsibility for constant approach of each other. And yet, in proximity all social 'settlement' is shattered, and we should not consider the pastor to be immune to proximity.

In this regard I want to trace what remains of the pastor's subjectivity when it is stripped of its pride and virility of consciousness and intentionality. As I have shown in Chapter 2, Emmanuel Lévinas asserts the irreducibility of actions of love whereby the self departs from itself 'gratuitously' and 'without return'. The doer or decision-maker 'gives' him- or herself and does not anticipate (in fact shuns) any gratitude and/or retrospective authorisation by the receiver (TTO: 345-359). The act of gift-giving is an ineluctably one-way act through which 'my ego is donation', a gift which goes to the other without 'returning' to the giver in the form of recognition and gratitude. Such actions indicate the possibility of a 'radical generosity' on the part of the giver: theirs is a one-way movement that goes out to the other human and does not return. They also indicate the possibility of a particularly heteronomous experience of the receiver by the giver as totally self-identical and already individualised other, i.e. as the vulnerable or 'naked' other. The giver is the messiah who takes it upon him or herself to act for the benefit of each unique other prior to thematising and comparing their needs. Unlike the pastor, the giver has no need for thorough knowledge of the other's needs and interests. I submit that the pastoral social role appropriates the more fundamental notion of subjectivity as 'my neighbour's keeper'. There is the *me* of the ethical command to be-for-my other - a command which is in place before my freedom so that *I am in no position*, pastoral or other, either freely to accept or to decline responsibility for my neighbour; to bestow meaning and time on the neighbour's sufferings or to ignore them. It is important that this 'me' be theoretically disengaged from the economical 'use' to which it is put by 'pastorship'. And perhaps forms of *ascesis* or exercises of the soul must also be found for the 'de-habitualization' of pastors and their subjects. We must trace the significance of our compassion beyond its politico-juridical delimitation and politicisation. We must feel free to donate compassion.

VI
Beyond formal-informal justice

Why is not proximity complete satiety, the most perfect stillness of contact, more perfect than the repose of the sleeping baby at its mother's breast. Why is proximity not a unity like the condition of the spherical double humans of Aristophanes' speech in Plato's *Symposium*? That it is not indicates that the proximate signifies or refers in the manner or mode of an absence. But the absence is not a lack: it is infinitely Absent, illeity, absent in an immemorial past (DEHH: 230).

Let me, in conclusion, do away with the dichotomy formal-informal justice. What is required, I argue, is a critique of 'formal' legal justice for its failure to uphold the significance of the obligation to be-for-each-other. The latter is not to be confounded with spatio-temporal contiguity but it is rather *a liberty* connected to the subject's ethical hypostasis; the being-for-the-other can only be expressed as the event in which the loneliness of the subject is shattered in the consciousness of being responsible for the other. The desired 'justice' must be such that it may allow its agents, including the most aloof of judges, to substitute themselves for-the-other, in pure emotion which they cannot withhold, and so to 'put themselves in the other's place'. But it must *also* be stressed that, as I have shown in other parts of this thesis, the ego's obligation to 'substitute itself' for its other is not fulfilled in 'empathy' for the other's circumstances but must remain non-sensical exposure to the *non-sense* that commands the being-for-each-other. Proximity thus induces an infinite restlessness in the ego, it is 'non-repose itself' (DEHH 230). The restlessness of the one-for-the-other continues even if the neighbour is as close as may be, in the most peaceful of suburban streets or in the activity of the market-place.

We must pursue a critical study of both the legal and 'para-legal' phenomena in ways that show all the above. To criticise the informalist discourse for 'naturalising' what is in reality the 'radically situated' subject is not enough. Nor is it enough to demonstrate how in both rights-discourse and in interests/needs-discourse there is absurd privileging of the subject of consciousness and of being-for-oneself over and above the subject of obsession and being-for-the-neighbour. Critics of informal justice help us to understand the deficiencies of this ill-theorised discourse and its reductionist assumption that proximity equals spatio/temporal and psychological contiguity. This *finite* representation of proximity in informal justice discourse opposes (but also 'complements' and replicates) the *ideality* of the formal legal presentation of subjectivity by means of law's supposedly '*immortal*' operations and 'immemorial' principles. Moreover, both 'formal' and 'informal' justice models centre around the idea of the individual as 'different' but also exchangeable (non-unique) subject of so-called 'transcendental' rights/interests, and member of a closed totality (family, community, *polis*, nation etc); at the same time, the individual's subjectivity-in-exile is 'excepted' from responsibility as compassion and gratuitous charity. Thus, the individual subject of care (be it the 'immortal' subject of juridical rights or the finite being of interests/needs) becomes - perversely - the subject which is 'excepted' from the possibility of emotions, alterity, charity and obsession as personal responsibility.

Informal justice discourse failed ethically in its attempt to ground justice in space and time. In so doing it added itself to the 'ideal' representations of subjectivity and proximity of the institution of formal law. In circumstances where society is governed as 'population' and where the regulation and the synchronisation of societal inter-*esse* involve even the most intimate bonds between subjectivity and itself or its 'similar' others, informal justice discourse adds a *material* sense of the human inter-*esse* (interests/needs) to law's most abstract sense. At the same time, ADR discourse 'extracted' from the ideal presentation of justice its element of time: informal justice, as we saw, retains from law a sense of urgency but despises its 'patience'. Informal justice practices are 'acted spontaneously', *not* endured. In this way informal justice discourse *complements* the ideal representation of subjectivity and proximity by law. The latter, left to its own devices at least, suffers a crisis. Ideality, at least, imagines an infinity. By now, litigants whom the state judge may judge unfairly will rarely have the consolation of faith in the promise of a final Day of Divine Judgment beyond; nor will the litigant who suffers delay be able to set this against the promise of infinity. With regard to the exclusion of proximity from the realm of positive, modern 'impersonal' law, the introduction of ADR discourse and practices is perhaps a 'spontaneous', i.e. irresponsibly obsessive attempt to soothe the symptoms of a crisis by abstracting the problem of proximity from the realm of the law altogether. But what is required, I submit, is an un-settlement of the assumptions that law makes with regard to proximity. It is important that we expose the judge who sits comfortably in the courtroom as someone confronted with an outrage. His courtroom is *from the start* 'occupied by' and 'at the disposal of' the anarchist other whose nakedness cannot be 'hidden' by rights or by interests/needs, except in absurd ways. The scandal can only be addressed by, and so 'clothed' with, the judge's own personal responsibility. Today, to the extent that the state judge is aided by the 'community mediator' (as 'pastor'), or by the disputants themselves (who 'take care for themselves'), it is even more urgent to profess our love - even if in a clumsy way - for a society in which there is 'no distinction between those close and those far-off', but in which there also remains the impossibility of passing-by the closest (AE: 158).

For it is 'only' in ethical proximity that justice remains justice.

Epilogue

The notion of ethical proximity, as employed in this thesis, points not only to humanity but also to society. The term 'society' refers to the horizontally structured associations in which we are known to be, and wish to be, in synchrony 'with each other', but also to those vertical associations of power, domination, control, which entail ethical violence, that is, the violence of abstracting my other from all its associations except with *me*. Horizontal associations stand for reciprocal relationships based on democratically regulated exchange: the process of commercial pacification synchronises and transforms into contract the violence and conflict to which the subject of needs and wants is driven. Violence and aggression are inherent in the idea of self 'with' others, all of whom are similar 'objects' of nature and fate, and subjects of innumerable needs/interests while being faced with scarce resources. 'Subjectivity', here, suggests an individual being as additive entity in a social totality; a being that is different from everyone else but is not unique. Its meaning - the 'essence' (or *esse*) of subjectivity - consists in 'perseverence' in participating in society and in *being for itself*. 'Society', in turn, is traced to beings' desire to 'be with each other' to the extent that this 'being-with' contributes to collective well-being. In Lévinas' terminology 'society', as the additive total of the multifarious individual beings' engagement in horizontal association, constitutes an 'inter-*esse*'.

Unlike commerce, democracy and exchange, the 'vertical' patterns of association (for instance the parent-child, teacher-student, doctor-patient, judge-judged relationship), in invoking a dimension of 'height' present us with a problem of justification. In this regard Max Weber has identified 'state power' as the 'monopoly of legitimate violence'. Prior to the French Revolution religious dogma and institutions had helped the state to retain this 'monopoly' mainly by legitimising state power and its violence in lending it powerful religious symbols which commanded faith. In modernity, however, this relationship disintegrates and the bureaucratic welfare democratic state faces a legitimation crisis. As sovereignty and the rule of law give way to new, modern, mechanisms for 'ordering' society, so the old religious symbols no longer command the same belief (*Glaube*) in the morality of state-backed 'one-way' actions and decisions: in such conditions, the social web suffers the results of a symbolic 'impoverishment' in the exercise of the power, mastery, and control necessary for 'vertical' associations.

In a society without religious symbolic dominance politics can only draw legitimacy from the idea of contract between individuals who are increasingly thought of as autonomous. Although a contract can always be doubted, we have found no other solution than the institution of constitutional rules for consulting the 'ordinary people', whose individual moral vocations seem to matter little. Here, 'politics' is understood as a system for the distribution of power, starting from a body of additive 'citizens', and its study is the study of the rules of the democratic process. Nowadays, democratically empowered, autonomous individuals are politicised in asserting for themselves the power to speak of their needs and interests beyond the abstractions of the legal categories of rights; in defying their doctors' incorrigibility; and withdrawing their 'intimate' associations and 'natural' conflicts from the reach of the state law. However today's belief in autonomy *only partly* compensates for the fact that religious symbolism no longer commands faith in the words of the father, king or messiah who professes the symbolic. This is because contract, by its very nature, can only be of 'administrative' use: like the code of traffic regulations, a binding contract allows us to conceive of a guaranteed order.

In political theory, just as in law, we are incapable of conceding that there is a truth beyond meaning in the way vulnerable humans associate. We are told to tolerate the 'different', but we are incapable of admitting that there may exist a truth beyond our individual convictions. Politics lessens the fear of violent death (for instance, in Hobbes) and of instability (in Macchiaveli): it endows institutions with a duration well beyond the scope of the ephemeral human life. However bereft of religious or 'ultimate' grounds, modern politics is thought in contract theory to be self-founded, which is to say, ill-founded. For in reality the 'vertical' relations of hierarchy cannot be produced reciprocally, but require strictly individuated 'one-way' actions. The question of what these one-way actions mean, and whence they derive their force and authority, is only more perplexing in post-religious times. In fact, it appears that few ask it nowadays. Many are happy to eliminate the role of individual subjectivity from the question of 'what justifies' vertical relationships, if not to forget altogether that such relationships continue to exist despite the lapse in authority, and matter enormously. For these, there is simply nothing but the necessity of presupposing, anachronistically, a social contract. Without such an anachronism, we are told, 'we would turn to murder'. Others are intent on solving the perennial political problem of how to rid our desire to be 'with each other' of power, mastery and control.

According to Kant the philosophy of religion emerges in response to the problem of 'fundamental evil', and revolves around three themes: first, the power of the symbolic; second, that the symbolic requires faith in the one who professes it; and third, that religion is expressed through a *community*, such as synagogue or agora/ecclesia. Whereas traditional sociology focused on symbolism and faith alone, contemporary consensus theories place equal emphasis on the third of the three themes. More specifically, the sociologies of Jürgen Habermas and the theory of justice of John Rawls recognise that the problem of legitimation of politics must no longer be put solely in terms of the law-sovereignty model of human association, but rather in terms of the kind of association that has succeeded religious communities. The sense of ecclesiastic congregations has been 'lost', and it is therefore no longer possible to justify the exercise of power through religion. In short, we are faced not only with symbolic nakedness and absence of faith, but with an equal impoverishment of the very meaning of modern 'community'. Separated from religion, community has no other function than to promote an abstract social coherence through 'solidarity', 'empathy' and the desire to 'communicate' with each other, which supposedly is shared by what otherwise are all-too-different individual beings. The model of the modern contractual and democratic political body thus emerges as the only alternative to the now-lost sense of multiple religious communities. Solipsism is avoided if democratic politics are justified by reference to an 'ethics of dialogue', which promotes constant confrontation of values and is supported by the rules of liberal constitutions. On the other hand, the sociology of Michel Foucault asserts the revival of 'religious' themes such as that of 'pastorship', which as I have shown haunts those who claim informal justice practices to be 'emancipatory', and warns of their inherent dangers.

Aristotle surely erred when he wrote that 'just conduct is a mean between committing and suffering injustice' (*Nichomachean Ethics* [1987: 163]). In my view just acts are a mean between committing 'ethical violence' and suffering responsibility for it. Through Lévinas' 'God-less' metaphysics we do not need anachronistically to suppose an origin of law and society in anything other than religion, nor to speculate, like the jurist Rawls and the sociologists Habermas and Foucault, about the demise or revival of religious types of community.

In his *La sagesse de l'amour* (1984; English transl. 1997), Alain Finkielkraut makes a comprehensive and admirable summary of Lévinas' philosophy; commenting on Lévinas' statement that the concept of the face is 'a fine risk to be run' (OB: 120), Finkielkraut observes that today the ethical encounter with the other 'shames' the modern subject's 'devastating dynamism and self-interested motives'. All in all:

Lévinas's originality consists not so much in his emphasis on morality, in the midst of a *political* century, as in his transposition of morality into a new schema. He locates Good not at the end, in the ... glorious future of historical fulfilment, but at the beginning, in the age-old experience of the encounter with Others. Not struggle but ethics becomes the fundamental meaning of Being for others. The face-to-face encounter ... evokes responsibility rather than conflict ... This does not mean that peace reigned before war, but that *ethical violence* precedes the contest between consciousness and the adversarial relation. The Good seizes me, holding on without my consent. I can disobey, but I cannot escape it (Finkielkraut 1997: 21).

This thesis has examined legal phenomena from the perspective of this transposed morality. In the matter of euthanasia and legal declarations for the withdrawal of life-support from comatose patients, the challenge is not to choose between the juridical representation of the patient as holding a right-to-die, or as being the subject/object of vital interests, but to trace the way in which decision-makers can 'mark' the patient with 'an identity of uniqueness'. In connection with sterilisation of the incompetent, what is at stake in the guise of the right to reproduce is the very right to become infinitely responsible for another human beyond the constraints set by nature or consciousness, in irreducible surprise. In another instance, the judicial policy of 'restraining' the exercise of patients' rights, under the justification of 'protecting' the highly moral and 'intimate' nature of the doctor-patient relationship from unnecessary litigation, apears as moral indifference to the non-sense of human suffering and the compassion it raises. Theories of biopolitics were shown to have a bearing on the issue of 'informed consent' of the modern, 'autonomously suffering' patient. Accepting the premise that in conditions of biopolitical exercise of power, there is no longer a rigid separation between private suffering and public well-being, I argue that the politico-juridical interest in 'biological being' also presupposes an attitude of moral indifference towards this being as neither finite being nor 'nothingness', but as 'subjectivity-in-exile'.

The task is to reclaim for the agent of justice the liberty to approach the other as unique - compassionately extracted from its natural and social circumstances - but not yet as 'abstract', since in proximity *qua* right to personal responsibility the unique 'other' is offered the materiality of the judge's 'emotion'. If modern law seems intent on projecting on the modern subject of consciousness the 'dynamism' and 'self-interested motivation' to do both good and evil (interchangeably); and if, thus, it fails to engage with the 'ethical violence' that controls the face-to-face, this thesis is an attempt to expose the irrepressible *shame* that this project entails. The moral indifference that modern law prescribes that its agents and subjects show towards ethical proximity is in itself a legal 'evil' and a 'sin', in the sense Lévinas gives these terms. Law cannot eradicate the obsessive compassion and the one-way acts of caring for the other being's absurd suffering that constitute the original deployment of social relations, although it does ignore them (in the sense that it proscribes reflection on these issues). As a result, I have claimed, modern law is plagued by the 'violence of irresponsibility' - that is, the concealment of responsibility for acts of 'ethical violence' (for instance, in masking the violence of human rights whereby the other is marked with an identity of uniqueness). In this *suppressed* form, responsibility and compassion manifest themselves only as bad conscience, 'sin' and 'shame', as 'responsibility' in spite of the refusal of responsibilities. This irresponsibility is not without real consequences. The reader will recall that in the event of the English judge who banned the enforced sterilisation of an incompetent adult woman, the recognition of the patient's 'inalienable' right to reproduce was couched in terms of false expectations of future recovery. As a result of this irresponsibility, I claimed, the above right (which, for me symbolises the right to become responsible for another human being non-intentionally) has become an empty reference for subsequent (contradictory) decisions, which nevertheless refer to the 'same' right as the precedent recognised in the abstract.

In order to move beyond these circumstances I have had recourse to Lévinas' *disinterest*, a semi-religious term which would be outmoded if Lévinas did not give it:

> an absolutely unexpected location ... [Lévinas'] language is Corneille's, [but] the plot is from Racine. And the same holds true for *agape* and *eros*, for the love of one's neighbour and for romantic love: 'No one is not good voluntarily [OB: 11].' It is not out of choice that we lose our heads, let our minds stray, cast prudence to the winds, reject the advantageous counsel and forethought of utilitarian reason ... [However, when] [s]tripped of our own initiative, our consciousness is bound [citing Maurice Blanchot:] 'fatally and as if against our will, for another who attracts us all the more because he seems to be outside the possibility of meeting because he is so beyond the scope of things that interest us' (Finkielkraut 1997: 22).

Elsewhere in the thesis I traced this location of disinterest in the theatrical origins of the western legal order. Aeschylus' *Oresteia* is useful in pointing out that our most ancient memory is not of death and mourning (the theme of *Antigone)* but of responsibility for the juridical 'exile' and political 'uprooting' of ethical subjectivity. That story is important in that it is more than a piece of mythical drama that can be re-enacted, for contains within it a 'counter-narrative' regarding the crucial function in the story of Orestes' 'proximities' whilst in exile in a *topos* which the play could not, and would not, represent. Between Orestes and the crucial but absent 'others' who absolved him involuntarily there is no 'theatre', but unmediated face-to-face. This story entails a *diachronic* truth: the *common* origins of love and law lie in the non-intentional, disinterested being-for-the-other. The other is approached *as* other: without name and distinguishing characteristics, beyond memory and representation, outside an economy of pain and pleasure, as non-thematisable as its 'sufferings'; and yet, thanks to the good violence of affectivity and obsession, the other is approached *as* unique. I argued that if the subject of law inside the *polis* exists, for law, only as essence, and in the form of an 'immortal' juridical *persona* (as fictional identity that has to be attached to), at the same time it is 'face-less: it is thought of as cut off from proximity or the face-to-face. It takes indifference towards the other to engage with him or her only as persona and not as face.

Alas I also showed, from the point of view of 'biopolitics', how it has happened that in the west the juridico-political order is established as if 'independent' of ethical proximity. Disinterest is denied responsibility: indeed we now think of disinterested, obsessive acts of kindness as if they were 'spontaneous' and therefore innocent of responsibility, or from a more sophisticated theoretical point of theory, as forms of radical irresponsibility. In *consequence*, such acts exists only in 'shame' or 'sin'. It is only because of this disorientation that the idea of 'my other' may today sound excessively 'abstract', and the idea of what I called the 'right to responsibility' appear to be a license for irresponsibility. That which in ethics is *my* abstract yet unique other is converted in biopolitics into an object of interests - as also, Giorgio Agamben argues, in the law-sovereignty model, which he claims correctly is inherently 'biopolitical'. In the latter, human life is 'excepted' from the sphere of normativity and of politics, and so is 'given over' to the gaze of biopolitical interest. In so far as it is biological life and being-for-itself, individual being can only attract interest. That interest alternates with indifference towards that which is inexpressible and 'useless' suffering, affectivity and responsibility. Whilst the transcendental ethical command to take each being as 'the only one that matters' continues, the absurd and non-sensical dimension of (its) sufferings is overlooked for the sake of focusing on essential needs. Thus, being becomes an *essentially unique* subject of biopolitical interest whilst the otherwise-than-being and essence is a matter of political indifference. Modern being is singular but also an additive member of a social totality, for instance under the gaze of a 'pastor' who attends to the individual needs of persons not 'for nothing' but for the sake of 'collective well-being'. It is my argument, finally, that it would be a mistake to try to complement the legal abstractions of subjectivity with the materiality of its 'tangible' interests, as in 'community mediation' and other 'informal justice' practices. This would only exacerbate the modern phenomenon whereby 'civil society' is thought of merely as 'commercial peace' and exchange between ego-centric beings, with its own determinism, *supposedly* outside the control of the responsibility of the one-*for*-each-other.

Bibliography

I
Works by Emmanuel Lévinas

AD   *L'Au-Delà du Verset*, 1982. Minuit, Paris.

AE   *Autrement Qu'être ou Au-Delà de l'Essence*, 1974. Martinus Nijhoff, The Hague.

BPW   *E. Lévinas: Basic Philosophical Writings*, 1996. A.T. Peperzak *et al*, eds., Indiana University Press, Indianapolis and Bloomington.

DE   *De l'existence à l'existant*, 1947. Vrin, Paris.

DEHH   *En découvrant l'existence avec Husserl et Heidegger*, 1974. 3rd ed., Vrin, Paris.

DF   *Difficult Freedom*, 1990. Transl. Seàn Hand, The Johns Hopkins University Press, Baltimore and London.

DL   *Difficile Liberté*, 1976. 2nd ed., Albin Michel, Paris.

DMT   *Dieu, la Mort et le Temps*, 1993. Grasset, Paris.

DVI   *De Dieu Qui Vient à l'Idée*, 1982. Vrin, Paris.

EaI   *Éthique et Infini*, 1982. Librairie Arthème Fayard, Paris.

EE   *Existence and Existents*, 1978. Transl. A. Lingis, Martinus Nijhoff, The Hague.

EN   *Entre-nous: Essais sur le Penser-à-l'Autre*, 1991. Grasset Paris.

HAH   *Humanisme de l'Autre Homme*, 1976. Fata Morgana, Montpellier.

LR   *The Lévinas Reader*, 1989. S. Hand ed., Blackwell, Oxford.

MT   *La Mort et le Temps*, 1991, Éditions L'Herne, Paris.

NP   *Noms Propres*, 1976. Fata Morgana, Montpellier.

OB   *Otherwise Than Being, or Beyond Essence*, 1981. Transl. A. Lingis, Martinus Nijhoff, The Hague.

OS   *Outside the Subject*, 1993. Transl. M. Smith, Stanford University Press, Stanford, California.

S   'La Substitution', 1968. *Revue Philosophique de Louvain* 66:487-508.

TaI	*Totality and Infinity*, 1969. Transl. A. Lingis, Martinus Nijhoff, The Hague.
TO	*Time and the Other*, 1987. Transl. R. Cohen, Duquesne University Press, Pittsburgh, Pennsylvania.
TTO	*The Trace of the Other*, 1986. Transl. A. Lingis in M. Taylor ed., *Deconstruction in Context*, University of Chicago Press.

II
Other works

Abel, R. L. 1973. 'A Comparative Theory of Dispute Institutions' in *Law and Society Review* 6 (2): 217-347.

Abel, R. L. ed. with intro. 1982. *The Politics of Informal Justice: The American Experience*, vol. 1, Academic Press, New York.

Aeschylus, 1926, 1930, 1956, 1952, 1957, 1963, 1983. *Agamemnon, Libation-Bearers, Eumenides, Fragments*, transl. H. Weir Smyth, H. Lloyd-Jones ed., Cambridge University Press, Cambridge.

Agamben, G. 1990. *La Communauté Qui Vient - Théorie de la Singularité Quelconque*, Seuil, Paris.

Agamben, G. 1997. *Homo Sacer. Le Pouvoir Souverain et la Vie Nue,* French transl. M. Raiola, Seuil, Paris.

Aristotle, 1987. *Nichomachean Ethics*, transl. J. E. C. Welldon, Prometheus Books, New York.

Austin, S. and M. K. Utne 1977. 'Discretion and Justice in Judicial Decision Making' in *Psychology in the Legal Process*, B. D. Sales ed., 163-209.

Back, N. *et al.* eds. 1984. *Health and Disease: A Reader*, Open University Press.

Baker, R. and M. A. Strosberg eds. 1995. *Legislating Medical Ethics - A Study of the New York State Do-Not-Resuscitate Law*, Kluwer Academic Publishers, Dordrecht, Boston, London.

Baross, Z. 1988. *The Scandal of Disease in Theory and Discourse*, Doctoral Thesis, University of Amsterdam.

Barthes, R. 1972. *Mythologies*, transl. A. Lavers, Noonday Press, New York.

Bataille, G. 1988. *Oeuvres Complètes: Hegel, la Mort et le Sacrifice*, vol. XII, Gallimard, Paris.

Bataille, G. 1989. *Theory of Religion*, transl. H. Hurley, Zone Books, New York.

Bauman, Z. 1991. *Morality and Ambivalence*, Polity Press, Cambridge.

Bauman, Z. 1992. *Intimations of Postmodernity*, Routledge, London.

Bauman, Z. 1992. *Mortality, Immortality and Other Strategies*, Polity Press, Cambridge.

Bauman, Z. 1993. *Postmodern Ethics*, Blackwell, Oxford.

Becker, C. 1975. 'Conflict and the Uses of Adjudication' in *Studies on Diversion*, the Law Reform Commission of Canada ed., Queen's Printer, Ottawa.

Benhabib, S. 1992. *Situating the Self-Gender, Community and Postmodernism in Contemporary Ethics*, Polity Press, Cambridge.

Berlin, I. 1969. *Four Essays on Liberty*, The Clarendon Press, Oxford.

Bermants, N. ed. 1976. *Psychology and the Law*, Vidmar, Toronto.

Bernasconi, R. and S. Critchley eds. 1991. *Re-Reading Lévinas*, Athlone Press, London.

Bernasconi, R. and D. Wood eds. 1988. *The Provocation of Lévinas*, Routledge, New York

Billig, M. 1988. *Ideological Dilemmas: A Social Psychology of Everyday Thinking*, Sage, London.

Billig, M. 1991. *Ideology and Opinions: Studies in Rhetorical Psychology*, Sage, London.

Blanchot, M. 1969. *L'Entretien infini*, Gallimard, Paris.

Blanchot, M. 1982. *The Space of Literature*, transl. A. Smock, University of Nebraska Press, Lincoln.

Blanchot, M. 1983. *La Communauté Inavouable*, Minuit, Paris.

Blanchot, M. 1986. *The Writing of the Disaster*, transl. A. Smock, University of Nebraska Press, Lincoln and London.

Blond, P. ed. 1988. *Post-Secular Philosophy - Between Philosophy and Theology*, Routledge, London and New York.

Bloor, M. and G. Horobin 1975. 'Conflict and Conflict Resolution in Doctor-Patient Interactions' in C. Cox and A. Mead eds., *A Sociology of Medical Practice*, Macmillan, London.

Boltanski, L. 1990. *L'Amour et la Justisse Comme Compétences. Trois Essais de Sociologie de l'Action*, Éditions Metailie, Paris.

Boorse, C. 1975. 'On the Distinction between Disease and Illness' in *Philosophy and Public Affairs* 5: 49-68.

Boorse, C. 1977. 'Health as a Theoretical Concept' in *Philsophy of Science*, 44: 542-571.

Boorse, C. 1987. 'Concepts of Health' in *Health Care Ethics*, D. van de Veer and T. Regan eds., Temple University Press, Philadelphia.

Bottomley, A. and J. Roche 1988. 'Conflict and Consensus: A Critique of the Language of Informal Justice' in R. Matthews ed., *Informal Justice?* Sage, London.

Boyd-White, J. 1985. *The Legal Imagination*, The University of Chicago Press.

Boyd-White, J. 1990. *Justice as Translation*, The University of Chicago Press.

Brazier, M. 1992. *Medicine, Patients and the Law*, 2nd ed., Penguin Books, Harmondsworth.

Brock, D. W. 1992. 'Quality of Life Measures in Health Care and Medical Ethics' in A. Sen and M. Nussbaum eds., *The Quality of Life*, Oxford University Press.

Brock, D. W. 1993. *Life and Death - Philosophical Essays in Biomedical Ethics*, Cambridge University Press.

Buchanan, A. B. 1991. 'The Physician's Knowledge and the Patient's Best Interest' in E. D. Pellegrino *et al.* eds., *Ethics, Trust and the Professions: Philosophical and Cultural Aspects*, Georgetown University Press, Washington D.C.

Burton, S. J. 1992. *Judging in Good Faith*, Cambridge University Press, Cambridge.

Cabe, J., D. Kallehen and G. Wiling 1994. 'Litigation and the Threat to Medicine' in *Challenging Medicine*, Taylor and Francis Books Ltd. London, chap. 3, 46-64.

Cadava, E. *et al.* eds. 1991. *Who Comes After the Subject?*, Routledge, London.

Campbell, C. S. and A. B. Lustig 1994. *Duties to Others*, Kluwer Academic Publishers, Dordrecht, Boston, London.

Cassell, E. J. 1979. 'The Subjective in Clinical Judgement' in Engelhardt, Jr. *et al.* eds., *Clinical Judgement: A Critical Appraisal*, Dordrecht, Holland, 199-215.

Cassell, E. J. 1991. *The Nature of Suffering and the Goals of Medicine*, Oxford University Press.

Chalier, C. 1984. 'Singularité Juive et Philosophie' in J. Rolland ed., *Emmanuel Lévinas*, Verdier, Lagrasse, 78-98 (espec. 96-97).

Childless, J. F. 1983. *Who Should Die? Paternalism in Health Care*, Oxford University Press, Oxford.

Ciaramelli, F. 1991. 'Lévinas' Ethical Discourse - Between Individuation and Universality' in R. Bernasconi and D. Critchley eds., *The Provocation of Lévinas*, Routledge, New York, chap. 5.

Cohen, R. ed. 1986. *Face to Face with Lévinas*, SUNY Press, Albany.

Cornell, D. 1991. *Beyond Accommodation: Ethical Feminism, Deconstruction and the Law*, Routledge, London and New York.

Cornell, D. 1992. *The Philosophy of the Limit*, Routledge, London and New York.

Cotterell, R. 1984. *The Sociology of the Law*, Butterworths, London.

Cover, R. 1986. 'Violence and the Word' in *Yale Law Journal* 95: 1601-1629.

Critchley, S. 1992. *The Ethics of Deconstruction. Derrida and Lévinas*, Blackwell, Oxford.

Daniels, N. 1988. *Am I My Brother's Keeper?*, Oxford University Press, Oxford.

Davies, M. 1996. *Textbook on Medical Law*, Blackstone, London.

De Cruz, S. P. 1988. 'Sterilisation, Wardship and Human Rights' in *Family Law* 18(6): 10-11.

Deflem, M. ed. 1996. *Habermas, Modernity and the Law*, Sage, London.

Deleuze, G. 1968. *Différence et Répétition*, Presses Universitaires de France, Paris.

Deleuze, G. 1977. *Dialogues*, Flammarion, Paris.

Deleuze, G. 1983. *Nietzsche and Philosophy*, transl. H. Tomlinson, Athlone Press, London.

Deleuze, G. 1984. *Kant's Critical Philosophy*, transl. H. Tomlinson and B. Habberjam, Athlone Press, London.

Deleuze, G. 1994. *Difference and Repetition*, transl. P. Patton, Athlone Press, London.

Derrida, J. 1978. 'Violence and Metaphysics' in *Writing and Difference*, Routledge, London and New York.

Derrida, J. 1981. *Glas*, Denoel/Gonthier, Paris.

Derrida, J. 1992. 'Force of Law: The Mystical Foundation of Authority' in M. Rosenfeld *et al.* eds., *Deconstruction and the Possibility of Justice*, Routledge, London and New York, 3-67.

Derrida, J. 1993. *Memories of the Blind: The Self-Portrait and Other Ruins*, transl. A Braul and N. Naas, University of Chicago Press.

Derrida, J. 1995. *The Gift of Death*, transl. D. Wills, The University of Chicago Press, Chicago and London.

Douglas, M. 1987. *How Institutions Think*, Routledge, London and New York.

Douzinas, C. and R. Warrington 1991. 'A Well-Founded Fear of Justice: Law and Ethics in Postmodernity' in *Law and Critique*, II(2).

Douzinas, C. and R. Warrington 1994. *Justice Miscarried - Ethics and Aesthetics in Law*, Harvester Wheatsheaf, New York.

Douzinas, C., R. Warrington and S. McVeigh 1991. *Postmodern Jurisprudence. The Law of Text in the Texts of Law*, Routledge, London and New York.

Dreyfus, H. L. and P. Rabinow 1982. *Michel Foucault - Beyond Structuralism and Hermeneutics*, Harvester Press, Brighton.

Durkheim, E. 1982. *The Rules of Sociological Method*, Macmillan, Basingstoke.

Dworkin, G. 1982. 'Autonomy and Informed Consent' in *Making Health Care Decisions: The Ethical and Legal Implications of Informed Consent in the Patient-Practitioner Relationship*, vol. 3, 'Appendices: Studies on the Foundations of Informed Consent', The President's Commission for the Study of Ethical Problems in Medicine and Biomedical and Behavioral Research, US Government Printing Office, Washington, D.C.

Dworkin, R. 1979. *Taking Rights Seriously*, 2nd ed., Duckworth, London.

Dworkin, R. 1986. *A Matter of Principle*, The Clarendon Press, Oxford.

Dworkin, R. 1993. *Life's Dominion: An Argument about Abortion and Euthanasia*, Harper Collins, London.

Ehrenreich, J. 1978. *The Cultural Crisis of Modern Medicine*, Monthly Review Press, London and New York.

Engelhardt, Jr *et al.* eds. 1979. *Clinical Judgement: A Critical Appraisal*, Dordrecht, Holland.

Epictetus, 1983. *Handbook of Epictetus*, transl. with intro. N. White, Huckett Publishing Co., Indiana.

Finkilekraut, A. 1997. *The Wisdom of Love,* transl. K. O'Neill and D. Suchoff, University of Nebraska Press, Lincoln and London.

Fish, S. E. 1971. *Surprised by Sin -The Reader in Paradise Lost,* University of California Press, Berkeley, LA.

Fish, S. E. 1980. *Is There a Text in This Class? The Authority of Interpretive Communities,* Harvard University Press, Cambridge, Mass.

Fish, S. E. 1989. *Doing What Comes Naturally: Change, Rhetoric and the Practice of Theory in Literary and Legal Studies,* Duke University Press, Durham.

Fish, S. E. 1994. *There's No Such Thing As Free Speech - And It's a Good Thing Too,* Oxford University Press, New York.

Fitzpatrick, P. 1988. 'The Rise and Rise of Informalism' in R. Matthews ed., *Informal Justice?* Sage, London.

Fitzpatrick, P. ed. 1991. *Dangerous Supplements,* Pluto Press, London.

Fitzpatrick, P. 1992. *The Mythology of Modern Law,* Routledge, London.

Fitzpatrick, P. 1993. 'Relational Power and the Limits of the Law' in *Law and Power: Critical and Socio-legal Essays,* K. Tupri *et al.* eds., Deborah Charles Publications, Liverpool.

Foucault, M. 1971. *Madness and Civilization,* Tavistock Press, London.

Foucault, M. 1974. *The Order of Things,* Tavistock Press, London.

Foucault, M. 1979. *An Inroduction, The History of Sexuality,* vol. 1, Allen Lane, The Penguin Press, London.

Foucault, M. 1980. *Power/Knowledge, Selected Interviews and Other Writings 1972-1977,* C. Gordon ed., Harvester Press, Brighton.

Foucault, M. 1980. 'The politics of Health in the Eighteenth Century' in *Power/Knowledge, Selected Interviews and Other Writings 1972-1977,* C. Gordon ed., Harvester Press, Brighton, 166-82.

Foucault, M. 1984. *The Foucault Reader,* P. Rabinow ed., Pantheon Books, New York.

Foucault, M. 1987. *The Use of Pleasure, The History of Sexuality,* vol. 2, Penguin Books, Harmondsworth.

Foucault, M. 1988. *Politics, Philosophy - Interviews and Other Writings 1977-1984,* L. Kritzman ed., Routledge, London and New York.

Foucault, M. 1988. *The Care of the Self, The History of Sexuality,* vol. 3, Penguin Books, Harmondsworth.

Foucault, M. 1994. *Michel Foucault: Ethics - The Essential Works 1,* P. Rabinow ed., Allen Lane, The Penguin Press, London.

Freeman, M. D. A. ed. 1988. *Medicine, Ethics and the Law,* Stevens, London.

Frug, M. J. 1992. *Postmodern Legal Feminism,* Routledge, London.

Gadamer, H.-G. 1996. *The Enigma of Health,* Polity Press, Cambridge.

Galanter, M. 1981. 'Reading the Landscape of Disputes: What We Know and Don't Know (and Think We Know) about our Allegedly Contentious and Litigious Society' in *UCLA Law Review,* 31(4): 4-71.

Gilligan, C. 1982. *In a Different Voice - Psychological Theory and Women's Development*, Cambridge University Press, Cambridge.

Glover, J. 1990. *Causing Death and Saving Lives*, Penguin Books, London.

Good, B. J. 1994. *Medicine, Rationality and Experience - An Anthropological Perspective*, Cambridge University Press.

Goodrich, P. 1986. *Reading the Law*, Blackwell, Oxford.

Goodrich, P. 1990. *Languages of Law: From Logics of Memory to Nomadic Masks*, Weidenfeld and Nicholson, London.

Goodrich, P. 1991. 'Psychoanalysis in Legal Education. Notes on the Violence of the sign' in *Semiotics and the Human Sciences*, R. Kevelson ed., vol. 2, Peter Lang, New York.

Goodrich, P. 1993. 'Fate as Seduction: The Other Scene of Legal Judgement' in *Closure Or Critique. New Directions in Legal Theory*, A. Norrie ed., Edinburgh University Press, 121.

Goodrich, P. 1995. *Oedipus Lex*, University of California Press, Berkeley.

Goodrich, P. 1996. *Law in the Courts of Love - Literature and Other Minor Jurisprudences*, Routledge, London and New York.

Goodrich, P. 1997. *Law and the Unconscious: A Legendre Reader*, transl. P. Goodrich, A. Schütz and A. Pottage, Macmillan, London.

Goodwin, W. and E. Bronfen eds. 1993. *Death and Representation*, The John Hopkins University Press, Baltimore and London.

Grubb, A. and D. Pearl 1987. 'Sterilisation and the Courts' *CLJ* 1987:46.

Habermas, J. 1971. *Knowledge and Human Interests*, transl. J. J. Shapiro, Beacon Press, Boston, Mass.

Habermas, J. 1979. *Communication and the Evolution of Society*, transl. with intro. T. McCarthy, Heinemann Educational, London.

Habermas, J. 1982. *Autonomy and Solidarity - Interviews with Jürgen Habermas*, ed. and transl. P. Pews, Verso, London.

Habermas, J. 1987. *The Theory of Communicative Action*, transl. T. McCarthy, Polity Press, Cambridge.

Habermas, J. 1990. *Moral Consciousness and Communicative Action*, transl. T. McCarthy, Polity Press, Cambridge.

Habermas, J. 1997. *Between Facts and Norms*, Polity Press, Cambridge.

Hamilton, J. 1976. 'Individual Differences in Ascriptions of Responsibility, Guilt and Appropriate Punishment' in N. Bermants ed., *Psychology and the Law*, Vidmar, Toronto.

Harvard Medical School, 1968. 'Harvard Report: A Definition of Irreversible Coma', *JAMA*.

Heidegger, M. 1961. *An Introduction to Metaphysics*, transl. R. Manheim. Doubleday Anchor, New York.

Heidegger, M. 1962. *Being and Time*, transl. J. Macquarrie and E. Robinson, Harper and Row, New York.

Heidegger, M. 1978. *Basic Writings*, Harper and Row, New York.

Heidegger, M. 1983. *Lettre sur l'Humanisme*, Aubier-Montaigne, Paris.

Heller, A. 1987. *Beyond Justice*, Blackwell, Oxford.

Herrnstein-Smith, B. 1992. 'Judgement after the Fall' in M. Rosenfeld *et al.* eds, *Deconstruction and the Possibility of Justice*, Routledge, London and New York, 211-231.

Hogarth, J. 1974. 'Alternatives to the Adversary System' in *Studies on Sentencing*, The Law Reform Commission of Canada ed., The Queen's Printer, Ottawa.

Hunt, A. and G. Wickham 1988. *Foucault and Law*, Pluto Press, London.

Husserl, E. 1964. *The Phenomenology of Internal Time-Consciousness*, transl. J. S. Churchill, Indiana University Press, Bloomington.

Husserl, E. 1970 and 1977. *The Crisis of European Science and Transcendental Phenomenology: An Introduction to Phenomenological Philosophy*, transl. with an intro. D. Carr, Northwestern University Press, Evanston.

Husserl, E. 1973. *The Birth of the Clinic, An Archeology of Medical Perception*, Tavistock Press, London.

Illich, I. 1976. *Medical Nemesis: The Expropriational Health*, Boyars, London.

Irigaray, L. 1993. *An Ethics of Sexual Difference*, transl. C. Burke and G. Gill, The Athlone Press, London.

Irigaray, L. 1993. *Je, Tu, Nous: Towards a Culture of Difference*, transl. A. Martin, Routledge, London and New York.

Jackson, D. S. 1988. *Law, Fact and Narrative Coherence*, Deborah Charles Publications, Liverpool.

Jarvis, S. 1998. *Adorno: The Dialectics of Enlightenment - A Critical Introduction*, Polity Press, Cambridge.

Kant, I. 1978. *Critique of Pure Reason*, transl. N. Kemp Smith, Macmillan, London.

Kant, I. 1993.*Critique of Practical Reason*, transl. L. White-Beck, Macmillan, London.

Kant, I. 1995.*Groundwork on the Metaphysics*, transl. H. J. Paton, Routledge, London and New York.

Kass, L. 1985. *Towards a More Natural Science*, Free Press, New York.

Keenan, T. 1997. *Fables of Responsibility - Aberrations and Predicaments in Ethics and Politics*, Stanford University Press, Stanford, California.

Kennedy, I. 1981. *The Unmasking of Medicine*, Allen and Unwin, London.

Kennedy, I. 1988. *Treat Me Right*, Oxford University Press, Oxford.

Kennedy, I. and A. Grubb 1994. *Medical Law - Text with Materials*, 2nd ed., Butterworths, London.

Keown, J. 1988. *Abortion, Doctors and the Law*, Cambridge University Press.

Kerenyik, K. 1966. *Die Mythologie der Griechen* [in Greek], Hestia, Athens.

Kleinman, A. 1988. *The Illness Narrative: Suffering, Healing and the Human Condition*, Basic Books, New York.

Komesaroff, P. A. ed. 1995. *Troubled Bodies - A Critical Perspective on Postmodernism, Medical Ethics, and the Body*, Duke University Press, Durham and London.

Kristeva, J. 1986. *The Kristeva Reader*, T. Moi ed., Columbia University Press, New York.

Kristeva, J. 1987. *Soleil Noir - Dépression et Mélancholie*, Gallimard, Paris.

Lamb, D. 1986. *Death, Brain Death and Ethics*, Croom Helm, London.

Law Commission, 1993. *Mentally Incapacitated and Decision-Making: A New Jurisdiction*, Law Commission Consultation Papers, no. 128, Law Commission, London, paras 3.19-3.35.

Lefort, C. 1986. *The Political Forms of Modern Society - Bureaucracy, Democracy, Totalitarianism*, ed. and transl. with an intro. J. B. Thompson, Polity Press, Cambridge.

Legendre, P. 1993. 'L'impardonnable - entretien avec Pierre Legendre' in *Le Pardon - Briser la Dette et l'Oubli*, O. Abel ed., Série Morales n.4., Éditions Autrement.

Lerman, L. 1984. 'Mediation of Wife Abuse Cases: The Adverse Impact of Informal Dispute Resolution on Women' in *Harvard Women's Law Journal* 7: 57-113.

Leyh, G. ed. 1992. *Legal Hermeneutics: History, Theory and Practice*, University of California Press, Berkeley, CA.

Lidz, C. *et al.* 1983. 'Barriers to Informed Consent', *Annals of Internal Medicine* 99: 539-543.

Lingis, A. 1989. *Deathbound Subjectivity*, Indiana University Press, Indianapolis.

Lingis, A. 1994. *The Community of Those Who Have Nothing in Common*, Indiana University Press, Indianapolis.

Luhman, N. 1986. *Love As Passion: The Codification Of Intimacy*, transl. J. Gaines and D. I. Jones, Polity Press, Cambridge.

Luhman, N. 1990. *Essays on Self-Reference*, Columbia University Press, New York.

Lyons, D. 1992. *Moral Aspects of Legal Theory. Essays on Law, Justice, and Political Responsibility*, Cambridge University Press.

Lyotard, J. F. 1983. *Le Différend*, Minuit, Paris.

Lyotard, J. F. 1993. *Moralités Postmodernes*, Galilée, Paris.

MacIntyre, A. 1991. *A Short History of Ethics - A History of Moral Philosophy from the Homeric Age to the Twentieth Century*, Routledge, London and New York.

Mason, J. K. 1989. *Human Life and Medical Practice*, Edinburgh University Press.

Mason, J. K. and R. A. McCall Smith 1994. *Law and Medical Ethics*, 4th ed., Butterworths, London.

Matthews, R. ed. with intro. 1988. *Informal Justice?* Sage, London.

McIntyre, A. 1967. *A Short History of Ethics*, Routledge, London.

McIntyre, A. 1988. *Whose Justice? What Rationality?*, Duckworth, London.

McLean, S. A. M. ed. 1996. *Contemporary Issues in Law, Medicine and Ethics*, Dartmouth, Aldershot.

McLean, S. A. M. and G. Maher 1983. *Medicine, Morals and the Law*, Gower, Aldershot.

McVeigh, S. and C. Douzinas 1992. 'The Tragic Body: The Inscription of Autonomy in Medical Ethics and Law' in *Law, Health and Medical Regulation*, S. McVeigh and S. Wheeler eds., Dartmouth, Aldershot 1-35.

Merleau-Ponty, M. 1964. *Phenomenology of Perception*, transl. P. Kegan, Routledge, London and New York.

Merquior, M. J. 1985. *Foucault*, Fontana Press, London.

Miller, R. and A. Sarat 1980-81. 'Grievances, Claims and Disputes: Assessing the Adversary Culture' in *Law and Society Review*, 15: 525-565.

Minson, J. 1986. *Genealogies of Morals - Nietzsche, Foucault, Donzelot and the Eccentricity of Ethics*, Macmillan, London.

Momeyer, R. W. 1989. *Confronting Death*, Indiana University Press, Indianapolis.

Murphy, T. 1991. 'The Oldest Social Science? The Epistemic Properties of the Common Law Tradition' in *The Modern Law Review*, 54: 2.

Murphy, T. 1998. *The Oldest Social Science*, Oxford University Press.

Nader, L. 1988. 'The ADR Explosion - The Implications of Rhetoric in Legal Reform' in *The Windsor Yearbook of Access to Justice* 8: 261-291.

Nordenfeldt, L. ed. 1994. *Concepts and Measurement of Quality of Life in Health Care*, Kluwer Academic Publishers, Dordrecht, Boston, London.

Nussbaum, M. C. 1996. *The Therapy of Desire - Theory and Practice in Hellenistic Ethics*, Princeton University Press.

O'Connor, N. 1991. 'Who Suffers?' in R. Bernasconi *et al.* eds., *The Provocation of Lévinas*, Routledge, New York, 229-233.

Papanikolaou, A. D. 1989. *Etymological Dictionary of Ancient Greek* [in Greek], University of Athens Press, Athens.

Pavlich, G. C. 1996. *Justice Fragmented: Mediating Community Disputes under Postmodern Conditions*, Routledge, London and New York.

Pease, A. and C. Fitzmaurice 1986. *The Psychology Of Judicial Sentencing*, Manchester University Press.

Pellegrino, E. D. *et al.* eds. 1991. *Ethics, Trust and the Professions: Philosophical and Cultural Aspects*, Georgetown University Press, Washington D.C.

Peperzak, A. T. 1993. *To the Other*, Purdue University Press, West Lafayette, Ind.

Peperzak, A. T. ed. 1995. *Ethics as First Philosophy - The Significance of Emmanuel Lévinas for Philosophy, Literature and Religion*, Routledge, London and New York.

Pichot, A. 1993. *Histoire de la Notion de la Vie*, Gallimard, Paris.

Podlecki, J. 1984. *The Political Background of Aeschylean Tragedy*, University of British Columbia Press.

Porter, R. ed. 1996. *The Cambridge History of Medicine*, Cambridge University Press.

Rabinow, P. ed. 1994. *Michel Foucault; Ethics; The Essential Works 1*, Allen Lane, The Penguin Press, London.

Rawls, J. 1973. *A Theory of Justice*, Oxford University Press.

Rawls, J. 1986. *Political Liberalism* (rev. ed.), Columbia University Press, New York.

Rawls, J. 1989. 'The Domain of the Political and Overlapping Consensus' in *New York University Law Review*, 64(2).

Rheinstein, F. 1954. *Max Weber on Law in Economy and Society*, Harvard University Press, Boston, Mass.

Ricoeur, P. 1966. *Freedom and Nature: The Voluntary and the Involuntary*, transl. with intro. E. V. Kohák, Northwestern University Press, Evanston, Illinois.

Ricoeur, P. 1975. *The Rule of Metaphor: Multi-disciplinary Studies of the Creation of Meaning in Language*, transl. T. Czerny, University of Toronto Press.

Rolland, J. ed. 1994. *Emmanuel Lévinas, Les Cahiers de la Nuit Surveillée*, Verdier, Lagrasse.

Rorty, R. 1989. *Contingency, Irony and Solidarity*, Cambridge University Press.

Rose, G. 1992. *The Broken Middle - Out of our Ancient Society*, Blackwell, Oxford.

Rose, G. 1996. *Mourning Becomes the Law - Philosophy and Representation*, Cambridge University Press.

Rosenfeld, M. *et al.* eds. 1992. *Deconstruction and the Possibility of Justice*, Routledge, London and New York.

Rothman, D. 1991. *Strangers at the Bedside: A History of How Law and Bioethics Transformed Medical Decision-making*, Basic Books, New York.

Rouland, N. 1988. *Anthropologie Juridique*, Puf, Paris.

Santos, B. De Sousa 1982. 'Law and Community: The Changing Nature of State Power in Late Capitalism' in *The Politics of Informal Justice: The American Experience*, vol. 1, R. Abel ed., Academic Press, New York.

Sarat, A. ed. 1992. *The Fate of the Law*, University of Michigan Press, Ann Arbor.

Sartre, J.-P. 1956. *Being and Nothingness: A Phenomenological Essay on Ontology*, trans. H. E. Barnes, Pocket Books, New York.

Scarry, E. 1985. *The Body in Pain*, Oxford University Press, Oxford.

Schauer, F. 1988. 'Formalism' in *The Yale Law Journal*, 97: 509-48.

Schutz, A. and T. Luckmann 1973. *The Structures of the Life-World*, transl. H. T. Englehardt Jr. and R. M. Zaner, Northwestern University Press, Evanston, Illinois.

Schwartz, M. A. and O. Wiggins, 1988. 'Scientific and Humanistic Medicine: A Theory of Clinical Methods: A Phenomenological View' in K. L. White ed., *The Task of Medicine, Dialogue at Wickenburg*, The Henry J. Kaiser Foundation, Menlo Park, CA, 137-171.

Scott, C. E. 1995. 'A People's Witness beyond Politics' in *E. Lévinas: Basic Philosophical Writings*, A.T. Peperzak *et al.* eds., Indiana University Press, Indianapolis and Bloomington.

Sen, A. and M. Nussbaum eds. 1992. *The Quality of Life*, Oxford University Press.

Sennet, R. 1990. *The Conscience of the Eye. The Design and Social Life of Cities*, Faber, London.

Shonholtz, R. 1988/9. 'Community as Peace-maker - Making Neighborhood Justice Work' in *Current Municipal Problems* 15: 3-30.

Shotter, M. 1984. *Social Accountability and Selfhood*, Blackwell, Oxford.

Silbey, S. and A. Sarat 1989. 'Dispute Processing in Law and Legal Scholarship: From Institutional Critique to the Reconstitution of the Juridical Subject' in *Denver University Law Review*, 66(3): 437-498.

Singer, P. 1995. *Rethinking Life and Death: The Collapse of our Traditional Ethics*, Oxford University Press.

Steinbock, B. and A. Norcross eds. 1994. *Killing and Letting Die*, Fordham University Press, New York .

Szasz, T. S. 1975. *The Ethics of Psychoanalysis*, Routledge, London and New York.

Taylor, M. ed. 1986. *Deconstruction in Context*, University of Chicago Press.

Timsit, G. 1991. *Les Noms de la Loi*, Puf, Paris.

Tomasic, R. 1982. 'Formalised Informal Justice - A Critical Perspective on Mediation Centres' in *Proceedings of the Institute of Criminology: Community Justice Centres*, L. Street ed., University of Sydney Press.

Toombs, K. S. 1988. 'Illness and the Paradigm of the Lived Body' in *Theoretical Medicine* 9: 201-226.

Toombs, K. S. 1990. 'The Temporality of Illness: Four Levels of Experience' in *Theoretical Medicine* 11: 227-241.

Toombs, K. S. 1992. *The Meaning of Illness, A Phenomenological Account of the Different Perspectives of Physician and Patient*, Kluwer Academic Publishers: Philosophy and Medicine, Dordrecht, Boston, London.

Turner, B. S. 1980. 'The Body and Religion, Towards an Alliance of Medical Sociology and the Sociology of Religion' in *Annual Review of the Social Sciences of Religion* 4: 247-86.

Turner, B. S. 1981. 'Weber on Medicine and Religion' in P. Kegan ed., *For Weber, Essays on the Sociology of Fate*, Routledge, London and New York, 177-99.

Turner, B. S. 1985. 'The Practices of Rationality, Michel Foucault, Medical History and Sociological Theory' in R. Fardon ed., *Power and Knowledge, Anthropological and Sociological Approaches*, Scottish Academic Press, Edinburgh, 193-212.

Turner, B. S. 1987. *Medical Power and Social Knowledge*, Sage, London.

Turner, B. S. 1992. *Regulating Bodies - Essays in Medical Sociology*, Routledge, London and New York.

Turner, B. S. 1995. *Medical Power and Social Knowledge*, 2nd ed., Sage, London.

Unger, R. M. 1983. *Critical Legal Studies Movement*, Harvard University Press, Boston, Mass.

Vasseleu, C. 1998. *Textures of Light - Vision and Touch in Irigaray, Lévinas and Merleau-Ponty*, Routledge, London and New York.

Veach, R. M. 1977. *Case Studies in Medical Ethics*, Harvard University Press, Cambridge, Mass. and London.

Weber, M. 1976. *The Protestant Ethic and the Spirit of Capitalism*, Allen and Unwin, London.

Weber, M. 1978. *Economy and Society*, 2 vols., University of California Press, Berkeley, CA.

Weber, M. 1980. *Basic Concepts in Sociology*, The Citadell Press, NJ.

Werhane, P. 1996. 'Lévinas' Ethics: A Normative Perspective without Meta-Ethical Constraints' in *E. Lévinas: Basic Philosophical Writings*, A.T. Peperzak *et al.* eds., Indiana University Press, Indianapolis and Bloomington, 63.

Whitbeck, C. 1996. 'Ethical Issues Raised by the New Medical Technologies' in S A. M. McLean ed., *Contemporary Issues in Law, Medicine and Ethics*, Dartmouth, Aldershot.

Williams, B. 1993. *Ethics and the Limits of Philosophy*, Fontana Press, London.

Wittgenstein, L. 1983. *Philosophical Investigations*, Blackwell, Oxford.

Zaner, R. M. 1964. *The Problem of Embodiment: Some Contributions to a Phenomenology of the Body*, Martinus Nijhoff, The Hague.

Zaner, R. M. 1991. 'The Phenomenon of Trust and the Patient-Physician Relationship' in E. D. Pellegrino *et al.*, eds. *Ethics, Trust and the Professions: Philosophical and Cultural Aspects*, Georgetown University Press, Washington D.C. 45-67.

Zaner, R. M. 1993. 'Illness and the Other' in G. P. McKenny and J. R Sande eds. *Theological Analyses of the Clinical Encounter*, Kluwer Academic Publishers, Boston and Dordrecht.

Zizioulas, J. 1985. *Being as Communion*, SVS Press, New York.

Index